Medical

Kirk A. Johnson

Medical Stigmata

Race, Medicine, and the Pursuit of Theological Liberation

To JoAnn,

Thank you for your Support!

Kirk

palgrave
macmillan

Kirk A. Johnson
Philosophy and Religious Studies
Seton Hall University
South Orange, NJ, USA

ISBN 978-981-13-4812-9   ISBN 978-981-13-2992-0   (eBook)
https://doi.org/10.1007/978-981-13-2992-0

Cover image: WIN-Initiative

This Palgrave Macmillan imprint is published by the registered company Springer Nature Singapore Pte Ltd.
The registered company address is: 152 Beach Road, #21-01/04 Gateway East, Singapore 189721, Singapore

For the Family.

Acknowledgements

Thank you to Gabriel Ertsgaard and Max Orsini for your copy editing work.

Contents

1

Introduction

Race-based medicine is the process pharmaceutical companies use to assign specific drugs to racial groups. The idea of race-based medicine asserts that racial groups are biologically different. Therefore, drugs, tailor-made for racial groups are the best means for efficacious treatment within minority populations. For example, let's use a headache as an ailment. If an African American, Hispanic, and white individual followed the practice of race-based medicine, they would need an African American, Hispanic, and white aspirin to alleviate discomfort. However, such racially coded aspirin is not beneficial because a headache is not innately different due to anyone's racial classification. Illnesses and diseases do not discriminate. When all individuals take the same aspirin, the time it will take to alleviate the pain may vary due to each individual's internal response to pain and medicine, but the reaction to the aspirin is not dependent on external traits.

Consequently, the use of race-based medicine fragments racial groups. Its use attributes behavioral traits, labels, stereotypes and diseases which can stigmatize minority groups. Also, it can lead to prejudice and discrimination in the clinical practice. Race-based medicine misconstrues the distinctions of race, ancestry and genetics by assuming

© The Author(s) 2019
K. A. Johnson, *Medical Stigmata*,
https://doi.org/10.1007/978-981-13-2992-0_1

that race alone is the marker of disease, which inaccurately influences scientific studies and research. Race-based medicine is not the way to solve prevalent diseases in racial groups. Health disparities can be alleviated by the awareness and acknowledgement of predispositions and socioeconomic inequities existing in minority groups. This book examines the ways in which race is an inaccurate proxy for basing therapeutic intervention and how race-based medicine undermine minority communities' health.

This chapter uses the methods of the history of medicine, law, politics, genetics, and sociology to explore the origins of race-based medicine through eugenics. Eugenics was influenced by French biologist Jean Baptiste de Lamarck and Charles Darwin. Francis Galton, Charles Darwin's cousin, created the word 'eugenics.' There were two schools of eugenics: positive eugenics and negative eugenics. Positive eugenics asserted human breeding should be controlled to produce genetically superior human beings. Negative eugenics asserted the improvement of humanity can only happen by eliminating or excluding genetically inferior human beings.

Charles B. Davenport, the Father of American eugenics, established and directed The Eugenics Record Office. Davenport redefined eugenics as "the science of the improvement of the human race by better breeding"[1] to accomplish eugenics "we apply science to the problems of a class-ridden and socially heterogeneous society."[2] Eugenic influencers were exclusively self-identified as "White," "Anglo Saxon," "Nordic," or "Caucasian," stressing the idea of their racial superiority. Davenport categorized Africans, African Americans, Indians, and indigenous tribes as "genetically unfit" or inferior because they were less intelligent and primal. Davenport's racial classification was the first official American categorization of races. Davenport's 1908 *Inheritance in Canaries* study influenced the idea of disease and intelligence being associated to certain racial groups,[3] which created the notion of race-based medicine. As a result, eugenics' ideology embraced sociomedical racialism, meaning diseases were classified and attributed to certain races.[4] Eugenic influence created social and racial classifications through pathology- specifically, African Americans with Sickle Cell Anemia (SCA) and Jews with Tay Sachs Disease (TSD).

To be clear, eugenics did not solely dehumanize African Americans and Jews. Slavs, Italians, Poles, Irish, Asians, Turks, and Greeks were included in socially unfit classifications. However, there was a particular paranoia of an American epidemic with individuals with SCA and TSD. SCA affects groups from Indian, Asian, Saudi Arabian and Mediterranean backgrounds, but SCA was deemed a "black disease" due to the medical science, medical literature, and anthropological eugenic influences. SCA was perceived as a plague brought by black people, but factually it provided immunity from malaria.

The fear of SCA lead to the notion of Jim Crow (separate but equal) medicine, which led to segregated blood banks by the American Red Cross in WWII.[5] Neurologist Dr. Isador H. Coriat alleged TSD nerve cells contained poison that was transmitted through Jewish mother's milk.[6] Due to the social fear of contagion from SCA and TSD, African Americans and Jews faced abuse through sterilization and other forms of population control, including birth control, marriage control, and immigration policies.

Chapter 2 uses the methods of medical anthropology, clinical ethics, studies of the physician-patient relationship, biology and sociology to explore the misappropriations of the black body, race-based medical experiments, consequences of misappropriating the black body and the black community's response to false associations and harmful treatment. The eugenic perceptions of the "black body" produced misappropriations and falsified theories of the anatomy and biology of black individuals. The ideologies of African Americans being "lesser than" or "inferior" transferred into the fields of anthropology, anatomy, and biology, creating myths of innate human differences. The understanding that black bodies were innately different produced the terms "black hardiness" and "black durability," which affirms blacks have the innate capacity to endure or tolerate extreme conditions or illnesses. It was thought the experience of slavery made African Americans evolve to be a people of great endurance and stamina.

Such ideologies asserted black skulls were so thick that the skull would bruise or break the slave-owner's hand if he punched a slave,[7] or that longer limbs and shorter trunks were the reason why blacks could run faster than any group. Black hardiness led to an infatuation with the black body that created unconscionable harm in the clinical practice. As a result, J. Marion Sims, the father of gynecology, performed painful procedures on slave women without anesthesia.[8] The US government conducted mustard gas experiments on blacks and Hispanics which caused immediate and severe eye injuries, burns, oozing sores and blistering on the face, hands, underarms, buttocks, and genitals, resulting in "lung damage, psychological disorders, cancer, asthma, eye problems, and blindness."[9] Sloan-Kettering Institute's Dr. Chester M. Southam injected over 180 black Ohio State Prison inmates with live human cancer cells to see how a healthy human body would react to cancer cells.[10] Such experiences remain in the psyche of the black community through a key means of communication called oral tradition. As a response to race-based experimentation and race-based medicine, slaves created black homeopathy, a medical system that offers herbal, botanical, traditional, psychological, and spiritual approaches to medicine.[11]

Chapter 3 uses the methods of history of medicine, genetics, clinical ethics, research ethics, pharmacology, studies of the physician-patient relationship and sociology to assess significant heart studies before BiDil, "the black heart failure drug." There are numerous problems with BiDil. The data out of BiDil's clinical trials were based on unclear data because there was no control group to prove the drug was efficacious. BiDil was a rushed drug, only taking five years to reach the market with insufficient research funding. BiDil costs three times more than any other drug in its class, which does not benefit African Americans who are socioeconomically disadvantaged.

The idea of BiDil medicalizes race, a nonmedical issue, and interprets, defines and treats race as medical a problem. This recreates stigmas, stereotypes, and projected behavioral traits that are rooted in eugenic ideas. Finally, self-identification of one's race has no contextual validity. That is, it is a poor proxy based on other people's perception, excludes people who cannot self-identify (i.e. multi-racial or bi-racial individuals), has no use related to research questions on ancestry, and does not reflect the descent and ethnic origin of individuals.[12] BiDil an overly priced "quick fix" is not an adequate solution to health inequities in minority communities.

Race is a myth. Therefore, race should not be a proxy for disease. We are all genetically similar. For example, human genomes, 3 billion base pairs spread across 23 chromosomes, are 99.9% similar to one another with 0.1% difference (3 million pairs) with a smaller selection of the 0.1% that provide the raw material for locating the source of difference.[13] A more practical means for alleviating health inequity is improving physician's cultural competency, empathy and awareness with a keen focus on diet and nutrition.

Chapter 4 uses the methods of theology, textual criticism, exegesis, eisegesis, black church history and a combination of biblical and medical narrative to examine race in biblical literature as a tool for minority patient empowerment. This chapter also considers examples of the black church and personal clergy role in health advocacy. Black theology analyzes the oppression of black people, affirms the personhood of black people, and advocates their social and political liberation.[14] Black theology as survival theology is a response to the labels of race and illness by liberating minority communities to participate and speak out against the stigma of racial disease. Black theology is a tool that demonstrates multiple black perspectives and experiences. In contrast, race-based medicine encourages a truncated look at black experiences. Race-based medicine does not look at the totality of the African American pathological experience. Rather, it irrationally uses drugs as an inadequate solution for health inequity.

Black theology advocates empowerment and justice for African Americans in race-based environments that are rooted in and thrive on oppression. Blacks replaced dehumanizing identifications of race-based medicine and biblical literature with the belief that they were created by the same God with equal value. Black theology condemns race-based medicine because it separates racial groups as different beings through the construction of race. Furthermore, black theology asserts it does not matter what skin color you are, for we are all human beings and come from the same God.

As a response to race-based medicine, I suggest scripture, specifically the illness narratives in the gospels, can be used as an effective aid. For example, I connect the biblical and medical narrative of the leper in Galilee (cf. Mark 1:40–45) being denied healing in the temple with blacks being denied healing in white hospitals. The "Jesus" role was filled by the Black Panther Party's People's Free Medical Clinics emphasizing "completely free health care for all black and oppressed people."[15] Also, I reflect on past and current black church health movements to continue the push for health equity in communities of color. As mentioned in Chapter 3, the patient-physician relationship and diet and nutrition are suggested ways to improve health in minority communities. However, the black church has a unique position, and therefore can create dialogue in medical, religious, and theological settings on how race-based medicine and health disparities affect minority communities and ways the black church can respond through biblical inspiration and church advocacy.

Notes

1. Stern, Alexandra. *Eugenic Nation: Faults and Frontiers of Better Breeding in Modern America*. Berkeley: University of California Press, 2005, 11.
2. Sussman, Robert W. *The Myth of Race: The Troubling Persistence of an Unscientific Idea*. Cambridge: Harvard University Press, 2014, 55.
3. Largent, Mark A. *Breeding Contempt: The History of Coerced Sterilization in the United States*. New Brunswick, NJ: Rutgers University Press, 2008, 48.
4. McBride, David. *From TB to AIDS: Epidemics Among Urban Blacks Since 1900*. Albany: State University of New York Press, 1991, 19–20.
5. Wailoo, Keith. *Drawing Blood: Technology and Disease Identity in Twentieth-Century America*. Baltimore: Johns Hopkins University Press, 1997, 150.
6. Reuter, Shelley Z. "The Genuine Jewish Type: Racial Ideology and Anti-Immigrationism in Early Medical Writing About Tay-Sachs Disease." *Canadian Journal of Sociology* 31, no. 3 (Summer 2006), 298.
7. Hoberman, John M. *Darwin's Athletes: How Sport Has Damaged Black America and Preserved the Myth of Race*. Boston: Houghton Mifflin, 1997, 176.
8. Fett, Sharla M. *Working Cures: Healing, Health, and Power on Southern Slave Plantations*. Chapel Hill: University of North Carolina Press, 2002, 151.

9. Smith, Susan L. "Mustard Gas and American Race-Based Human Experimentation in World War II." *Journal of Law, Medicine & Ethics* 36, no. 3 (Fall 2008), 518.
10. Washington, Harriet A. *Medical Apartheid: The Dark History of Medical Experimentation on Black Americans from Colonial Times to the Present.* New York: Doubleday, 2006, 252.
11. Covey, Herbert C. *African American Slave Medicine: Herbal and Non-Herbal Treatments.* Lanham: Lexington Books, 2007, 42.
12. Whitmarsh, Ian, and David S. Jones. *What's the Use of Race? Modern Governance and the Biology of Difference.* Cambridge, MA: MIT Press, 2010, 128.
13. Wailoo, Keith, Alondra Nelson, and Catherine Lee. *Genetics and the Unsettled Past: The Collision of DNA, Race, and History.* New Brunswick, NJ: Rutgers University Press, 2012, 16.
14. Sanders, Cheryl J. "European-American Ethos and Principlism: An African-American Challenge." *On Moral Medicine: Theological Perspectives in Medical Ethics*, edited by Stephen E. Lammers and Allen Verhey, Wm. B. Eerdmans, 2012, 78.
15. Nelson, Alondra. *Body and Soul: The Black Panther Party and the Fight Against Medical Discrimination.* Minneapolis: University of Minnesota Press, 2011, 4.

2

Race-Based Medicine

Race-based medicine (RBM) or race-specific medicine asserts that race, understood as a biological reality and isolated from structural dynamics of discrimination, is the primary indicator for the predispositions of certain diseases. RBM is not a groundbreaking concept, but a recycled idea based out of the eugenics movement. Eugenics promoted specific social policies, ideologies, and biological classifications we ought not revive in the twenty first century. Sickle Cell Anemia (SCA) a non-fatal disease primarily (but not exclusively) affecting Africans and African Americans was the first hereditary disease examined in the eugenics era with Tay Sachs disease (TSD) to follow.[1] The father of RBM, Linus Pauling (1901–1994), was a key figure in the eugenic era. He officially identified SCA as a black person's disease, while also creating and revolutionizing molecular biology. This chapter will examine the roots of RBM through eugenic influences and how eugenics socially affected minority communities who possessed SCA and TSD.

© The Author(s) 2019
K. A. Johnson, *Medical Stigmata*,
https://doi.org/10.1007/978-981-13-2992-0_2

Eugenic Origins

In the early nineteenth century, French biologist Jean Baptiste de Lamarck (1744–1829) formulated his cornerstone theory of inheritance of acquired characteristics called Lamarckism, which affirmed, "environmental forces, both favorable and unfavorable, could alter human heredity and be transmitted down the familial line."[2] Lamarck's theory influenced Robert Knox's Races of Man (1850), Arthur Gobineau Essai's *sur l'inegalite des races humaine* or *The Inequality of Human Races* (1853) and Friedrich Max Muller's idea of an Aryan race (1853).[3] Lamarck's idea was embedded in the belief of degenerationism, which focused on the development of vestigial organs (i.e. tailbone and wisdom teeth). On an important note, a similar theological view of degenerationism called polygenism was prevalent around the sixteenth century. Polygenism suggests the human race has descended from two or more ancestral types. I will discuss polygenism in detail in chapter four. Degenerationism raised the fear that certain organs will lose their function and structure by each passing generation. Lamarck's most influential follower was Neo-Lamarckian Charles Darwin.

On November 24, 1859, English naturalist Charles Robert Darwin's book *The Origin of Species* quickly became a significant work of modern biological theory. He stressed the use, neglect and deterioration in organ development, including how the environment acts directly on organic structures. The two key theories from Darwin's work were evolution and natural selection. Evolution is a biological theory suggesting that all types of living beings have their origin in other preexisting beings, and that distinguishable differences resulted from modifications in successive generations. Natural selection is the process that results in the adaptation of an organism to its environment by means of selectively reproducing changes in its genotype, or genetic constitution. Evolution and natural selection were the foundational tools in the development of Social Darwinism.

However, the idea of "might makes right" preceded Origin.[4] Surprisingly, the "survival of the fittest" ideology did not come from Darwin, but from social philosopher Herbert Spencer, who created the phrase in 1864 and professed, "This survival of the fittest, which I have here sought to express in mechanical terms, is that which Mr. Darwin has called 'natural selection,' or the preservation of favoured races in the struggle for life."[5] Spencer's idea was adopted into Social Darwinism and developed into its own influence and interpretation for racial survival. Through Social Darwinism, it was unethical to help the weak because such actions aid the survival and reproduction of the "less fit," which threatens the progress and survival of the strong and equipped. Social Darwinism asserted the strongest or the fittest should flourish in society. Darwinism brought the idea to a level of unprecedented consciousness. Darwin made his mark on biology, but it is equally fitting to point out that Spencer was a huge voice in the late nineteenth century. Spenser's ideology advocated the natural evolution of groups and individuals to a higher level, from generation to generation, without any interference by any institution. Spencer sold over one million books in his lifetime.[6]

Darwin and Spencer's theories set the foundation for an emerging movement that would change the concept of American life called Eugenics. Eugenics is the belief in or study of the possibility of improving the qualities of the human species or a human population. Its creator Francis Galton, Charles Darwin's cousin, developed the phrase Eugenics, formally called "Race Hygiene," in 1883; Eugenics in the Greek "eu" (well or good) and "genesis" (to come into being, be born).[7] Galton believed the control and breeding of humans was a possible goal using statistics. In the Macmillan's Magazine and the book Hereditary Genius, Galton defended his stance for nature over nurture.[8] He spent his next forty years of life advocating the use of eugenics in society.

Galton stressed the concept of eminence for a better society. Eminent individuals are groups possessing high-ranking, distinguished, or prominent socioeconomic statuses in society. Eminent pedigree had to do with environment, culture, and education. In Galton's mindset, eminent humans produce more eminent humans and vice versa for "mediocre" humans. Galton used the 1865 edition of Dictionary of Men of the Time and obituaries to record the eminence of individuals. Galton, "estimated that 1 in 4000 men in Britain qualified as eminent. Close relatives of the eminent are much more likely to be eminent than are distant ones."[9] Galton continued his statistical work with his pupil Karl Pearson.

Along with his mentor, Karl Pearson revived Austrian monk and botanist Gregor Mendel's hereditary laws by a developed "biometrical" approach. Mendel created the theory called "unit characteristics" (now called genes by his research) with peas in his monastery's garden. Mendel believed genes did not go through different stages, but genes are transferred as separate and distinct units from one generation to the next.[10] Mendel's research resulted in his conclusion that planting two tall plants will produce a tall plant and the same result will happen with short plants. Furthermore, he assumed a tall and short plant would produce an average size plant, but to his surprise a tall plant was produced. Mendel's observations concluded some genes were dominant and some genes were recessive, which led to his famous 3:1 ratio producing thousands of variations of short peas. Mendel's findings resulted in a different approach to eugenics. Instead of the exclusive statistical approach for hereditary superiority (Galton), Mendel's experimental breeding was another means to do eugenic work.

Pearson partnered with Cambridge biologist Walter F. R. Weldon to continue Galton's research efforts. Pearson and Weldon had a total of fourteen years of work together, which resulted in one hundred published scientific papers, the production of the journal *Biometrika* promoting biometrical approaches, and the reconciliation of Galton's statistics and eugenics. Pearson and Weldon's professional partnership helped Galton to open Britain's Eugenics Record Office (BERO)[11] and an endowed research chair in eugenics at the University College London, in 1904. Galton promoted eugenic influence by the founding of The Society of Race Hygiene (1905), and the British Eugenics Society (1907).[12]

Darwin, Spencer, Galton, Pearson, and Weldon's work produced two schools of eugenics: positive eugenics and negative eugenics. Positive eugenics asserted human breeding should be controlled to produce genetically superior human beings. Negative eugenics asserted the improvement of humanity can only happen by eliminating or excluding genetically inferior human beings.[13] Galton was a positive eugenicist. Negative eugenics was more accepted in theory and practice in the United States, which became the blueprint for the German Eugenics Movement influencing the justification of the Holocaust. American geneticist and zoologist Charles B. Davenport visited London and dined with Galton, Pearson, and Weldon.[14] The meeting dramatically changed Davenport's ideologies of biology. His book, *Statistical Methods with Special Reference to Biological Variation*, was primarily influenced by Galton and Pearson. Davenport's encounter with the founding fathers of eugenics changed American social policy and biology in the early twentieth century and established Davenport as the father of American eugenics.

Davenport's influence in America was unrivaled. In 1904, Davenport received a grant from the Andrew Carnegie Institution to establish and become director of the Station of Experimental Evolution at Cold Harbor on Long Island, which performed breeding experiments on animals and plants.[15] Specifically, he focused on genetic make-up of family pedigree differing from Galton who focused on external characteristics. Through his grant, Davenport developed a record of families by sending surveys and questionnaires to public institutions (i.e. high schools, colleges, and churches). He received hundreds of survey results, from which Davenport concluded, "insanity, epilepsy, alcoholism, pauperism (poor/poverty), and especially feeblemindedness (mental incompetence or deficiency) were all hereditary conditions."[16] His goals for eugenics progressed to a wider scale as he mapped out the genetic health of the entire United States.

In 1909, Davenport met with psychologist Herbert H. Goddard (the first translator of the Binet-Simon intelligence tests into English) and encouraged Goddard to read British biologist (and creator of the Punnett Square) R. C. Punnett's 1909 book Mendelism. The Binet-Simon intelligence tests were developed by French physicians Alfred Binet and Theodore Simon to evaluate which children needed assistance in class. Davenport convinced Goddard that feeble-mindedness in children and other inherited conditions were caused by "unit characteristics" (genes) traced by family genealogy. The Binet-Simon intelligence test was influential in American standardized testing structure and the skewed procedure that characterized individuals with mental difficulties defined by eugenics.

In 1910, Davenport, with the aid of a huge donation from the widow of a railroad tycoon E. H. Harriman, established and directed

The Eugenics Record Office (ERO) with Harry H. Laughlin as super-intendent. The ERO instantaneously became the mecca for eugeni-cists, eugenics research, social policy, publication, and propaganda. In 1911, Davenport redefined eugenics as, "the science of the improve-ment of the human race by better breeding"[17]; to accomplish eugenics, "we apply science to the problems of a class-ridden and socially heter-ogeneous society."[18] After Davenport and Laughlin, there were many eugenicists who shaped American and European culture like Irving Fisher (founder of the American Eugenics Society), Margaret Sanger (founder of the Planned Parenthood Movement), Alfred Ploetz (founder of German Eugenics), Eugen Fischer (German eugenic anthropologist), and Fritz Lenz (German race hygienist).[19]

Eugenic influencers were exclusively self-identified as "White," "Anglo Saxon," "Nordic," or "Caucasian," stressing the idea of their racial superiority compared to other externally different groups or races. Davenport categorized Africans, African Americans, Indians, and Indigenous tribes were "genetically unfit" or inferior because they were less intelligent and primal. He also concluded that racial intelligence was absolute:

> In their mental traits… different peoples are unlike. It has formerly been maintained that the obvious mental differences in races are due to dif-ferences of education and training merely, but the experience with native tribes in Australia and Africa has shown that the children of these people do not respond in the same way as the white children to the same educa-tion… [T]he army intelligence test… showed that there is a marked dif-ference in average mental capacity between the major races of mankind, and even between the peoples of different parts of Europe… In fact, it seems probable that in the same country we have, living side by side per-sons of advanced mentality, person who have inherited the mentality of their ancestors of the early Stone Age, and persons of intermediate evolu-tionary stages.[20]

Davenport's racial classifications, which created the first official American categorization of races, determined the school you went to, what cemetery you would be buried in, where you lived, your fertility control, and who you married, which created the first official American categorization of races.[21] Davenport even influenced, The United States Office of Management and Budget (OMB). OMB constructed the racial and ethnic categories used to collect, organize, and analyze the country's demographic data. Davenport's work—which combined his classification of race combined with his interests in Mendelism—suggested that race not only affected intellectual ability, but also human ailments and diseases (i.e. hemophilia and Huntington's chorea).[22] His findings were based on his 1908 *Inheritance in Canaries* study,[23] which influenced the idea of disease and intelligence being associated to certain racial groups.

Eugenics has informed therapeutic intervention toward diseases and illnesses that are prevalent in specific minority groups. RBM has the same principle. Eugenics ideology (and later continued through RBM) embraced what Dr. David McBride called sociomedical racialism; diseases were classified and attributed to certain races.[24] Through eugenics justification, diseases and illnesses associated with certain racial groups should be treated because not only the disease affects that specific group, but it affects the entire society's environmentalism. Environmentalism, in this context, means the "social neutrality of infectious microbes, maintaining that immediate living conditions, employment experiences, dirt, and availability of health care were the primary determinants for the variation of disease rates among blacks and whites."[25] Eugenic influence created social and racial classifications through pathology.

In the early twentieth century, eugenic perceptions of African Americans as genetically unfit, inferior, and mentally incompetent resulted in a constructed perception of black folks as a national health threat. Eugenic concepts were used to influence disease diagnosis on a racial, biological and political landscape. Eugenics left African Americans associated with the "socially unfit": criminals, insane, alcoholics, feeble-minded, constitutionally weak, paupers, epileptics, deaf and blind, deformed, and individuals with specific diseases like SCA.[26] To be clear, eugenics did not solely dehumanize African Americans. Slavs, Italian, Polish, Irish, Asian, Turk, Hispanic, Greek and Jewish groups were included in socially unfit classifications. For the sake of race-specific diseases within minorities, SCA among African Americans and TSD among Jews will be the focus of this chapter. It is important to acknowledge the medical axioms of Tuberculosis (TB), Syphilis, Malaria, Diphtheria, Pneumonia, and Typhoid fever affected African Americans in American public health.[27] Yet, the first disease to influence racialized medicine was SCA.

Sickle Cell Anemia

The *A.D.A.M. Medical Encyclopedia* states SCA is caused by an abnormal type of hemoglobin; a protein inside red blood cells that carries oxygen. SCA falls under hematology which is the study of blood and blood diseases. Before any Western recognition of the disease, Indigenous African tribes had different descriptions of SCA symptoms using phrases like, "the Ga tribe's *Chwechweechwe,* the Fante tribe's *Nwiiwii,* the Ewe tribe's *Nuiduidui,* and the Akan tribe's *Ahotutuo.*"[28] The Ga, Fante, Ewe, and Akan tribes are based out of Ghana. These phrases were used to describe the continued distressing pains caused by SCA. Africans were concerned about the disease and the chronic pain SCA caused to fellow tribe members. In contrast, Western culture was more concerned with SCA as a public health concern for the well-being of those individuals eugenically and socially accepted. In the early twentieth century, American medicine rediscovered SCA through Dr. James B. Herrick.

On September 5, 1904, a twenty-year-old Grenadian dental student, Walter Clement Noel was rushed to Chicago's Presbyterian Hospital with respiratory problems. James B. Herrick, MD and his intern Ernest E. Irons, MD were on call. Irons took blood samples that had, "many pear shaped and elongated forms – some small."[29] Irons showed Herrick the unique examples of the blood smear. To his surprise, Herrick continued to monitor Noel for the next few years. Late 1905, Herrick uncovered German Pathologist M. Lowit discovery of odd shaped cells he called *sichelformiger* or sickle-shaped in appearance.[30] In 1909, Hematologist Russell L. Haden was the first to interpret SCA as a form of anemia and not a new blood disease. A step behind Haden, Herrick later used Lowit's terminology in the November 1910 issue of *Archives of Internal Medicine*, which made Noel's case the first recorded and documented case of SCA. Herrick deemed SCA unsolved after his publication, which did not stop the curiosity regarding SCA in the medical community.

In 1911, Benjamin Earl "B.E." Washburn wrote about SCA in the February issue of the journal *Virginia Medical Semi-Monthly*. Washburn reported about a patient Ellen Anthony at the University of Virginia Hospital with unusual looking blood cells. Washburn's report was the second reported case of SCA. The study and interest of SCA was growing modestly within the medical community and society. The concern was a result of the fear of a pandemic, rather than concern for the health and wellness of African Americans who were viewed as "less genetically fit." The future of America depended on the understanding and controlling the Black health threat. This idea that came from health statistician Fredrick L. Hoffman in his 1896 study *Race Traits and Tendencies of the American Negro* and *The Surgical Peculiarities of the Negro* by surgeon Rudolph Matas, which were the, "standard references for medical and sociological research through World War I postulating race distinctions as the basis for the black–white health discrepancy."[31] Hoffman's work advanced an ideology that race was the cause of health disparities, which influenced Davenport's racial and hematological classifications.

Davenport established distinctions within citizenship and racial categories. However, Viennese doctor and Nobel laureate Karl Landersteiner around 1901 established blood types A, B, O, M, N, and MN.[32] These blood characteristics were used to phenotypically classify "races" or "nationalities" as unique populations or expressions of their particular blood group. Landersteiner's discovery influenced Anatomic-genetics which came from the Mendelian tradition, emphasizing the importance of physiology and genetics within the black–white disease disparity. Genetic race traits were the basis for differing black and white disease mortality patterns.

In 1915, Major Robert W. Shufeldt of the USA Army Medical Corps published *America's Greatest Problem: The Negro*. Shufeldt's study produced research that suggested the inferiority of black folks. He felt social and economic equality for blacks were not important, but the health issues that would be created by the black community was a top priority:

The gravest problem to be faced in dealing with the…. Negro is not his or her industrial future or right to social equality with the white man or woman. It is the danger to the public of his or her contagiousness and infections from the standpoint of physical and moral disease.[33]

Shufeldt did not define himself as a eugenicist, but his idea of African Americans and their health was exactly aligned with eugenic principles. Hoffman, Matas, and Shufeldt were among numerous influencers in encouraging race-specific initiatives to treat African Americans in the public health sector of the early 1900s. For example, in the 1910s Henry Hazen and in the 1920s Henry R. M. Landis focused on TB among African Americans. Also, in the 1920s J. H. Masum Knox brought awareness to pediatric epidemiology for African American children.[34] Race-specific interests were developing ideas that race and disease were synonymous with each other. Ironically, Hoffman's, Matas', and Shufeldt's influence in minority specialization was not a form of beneficence (doing good) toward minority patient care, but an eugenic act to prevent a pandemic crisis caused by the Negro.

The technique that heightened targeted disease classification toward race was Victor Emmel's blood test. In 1916, Victor Emmel, an anatomist at the University of Washington, created a blood technique that was a central method for identifying and detecting sickled cells. SCA affects groups from Indian, Asian, Saudi Arabian and Mediterranean backgrounds,[35] but SCA was deemed a "black disease" due to the medical science, medical literature, and anthropological eugenic influences. SCA was perceived as a plague brought by black people, but factually it was immunity toward malaria. Since SCA was viewed a disease exclusively possessed by African Americans, individuals with SCA were instantly categorized as black. Emmel's test was used to justify Eugenicist Walter A. Plecker's "One Drop Rule," meaning one drop of Negro or Black blood makes you Black. After 1917, SCA changed from a clinical identity to a technological one.[36] Emmel's test meshed race and disease with identity.

Most doctors in the 1920s and 1930s who used Emmel's test assumed that blood and race were equivalent. The tendency for blood to sickle (meaning the red blood cells are shape like a crescent) was defined by Virgil P. Sydenshicker (1923) a latent disease quality present in "Negro Blood." Sydenshicker was from the University of Georgia Medical Department and characterized sickling in two forms: active and latent. Active sickling was characterized by anemia joint pain, muscle pain, and severe abdominal discomfort with leg ulcers. Latent was characterized with no symptoms of anemia, but had rare rheumatic attacks and abdominal pain.[37] John Hopkins physician John Huck (1924) defined sickling in three groups. First, a symptomless person had blood cells sickled after 24 hours with no symptoms. Second, a mild person occasionally had symptoms. Third, a severe person rarely became symptom free.[38] Until the 1950s, it was believed a person with SCA could go from one group or stage to another.

Emmel's test was used to search for "Negro Blood" and ancestry, which continued the racial thinking of eugenic racial origins and illness. Individuals characterized as "white" had SCA, but for them the classification was different. Sickling for whites was not a matter of illness, but a question of racial purity.[39] The consequence of being white with SCA was the stigma of being associated with "blackness;" socially outcaste and medically contagious. The stigma of "Negro Blood" permeated well into the mid-twentieth century. A June 1942 editorial by the New York Times called "Blood and Prejudice" reported the American Red Cross (ARC) segregated the blood donated by blacks and whites.[40] Under the ARC' "Negro Blood" and "non-Negro Blood" policy, the ARC labeled bags of blood by racial distinction and separated them for transfusions.[41] Such eugenic blood ideology was counterproductive in the World War II era.

The notion of Jim Crow Medicine (separate but equal) in a time of war demolished national solidarity and civic engagement. The white soldier died because "White Blood" ran out and he refused to receive "Negro Blood" or a black soldier could only receive "Negro Blood" without any other option. Eventually, the ban was removed. Emmel's test created an uncomfortable ambiguity regarding the external concept of racial identity. It awakened for society that the concept of race was not solely black and white. The variables are historical, geographical and literally skin deep at the cellular level.

Emmel's blood test of SCA complemented Mendelism to create racial identities and endorsed eugenics' role in society toward race and social policies. From the concepts of eugenics to Emmel's test, race was the crucial factor in disease discourse. Ironically, the idea of race did not influence medical science. Rather, medical science influenced ideas of race and social policies. In fact, the eugenic concepts of "Negro Blood" shaped insurance and social policies.[42] Medical science was the authority in shaping social policies in the early twentieth century, which maintained the status quo of race relations and developed the status of biological citizenship for African Americans with or without SCA.

Biological citizenship, termed by Dr. Adriana Petryna, means that, "the damaged biology of population has become the grounds for social membership and the basis for staking citizenship claims."[43] Eugenic influence created a racial and biological caricature of African Americans with and without SCA. Individuals with SCA were called a derogatory term "sickler." As a result, biological citizenship for African Americans was a social and racial contagion, which created stigmas like criminality, poor moral virtue and contagiousness that marginalized and symbolically expatriated African Americans through sterilization, population control, marriage control, and immigration policies.

Sterilization

ERO's Superintendent Harry H. Laughlin was the father of the eugenic sterilization and restrictive immigration policies in the early twentieth century. *Encyclopedia Britannica* describes sterilization, "as any process, physical or chemical, that destroys all forms of life, is used especially to destroy microorganisms, spores, and viruses." Sterilization was initially meant for the mentally ill or "feebleminded" individuals In 1897, Michigan state lawmakers considered House Bill No. 672, which proposed sterilizing feebleminded individuals through male castration and female ovariotomies.[44] The Bill was introduced by Congressman and Physician W. R. Edgar, but was defeated. In 1907, eugenics supporter US President Woodrow Wilson helped Indiana to adopt legislation making sterilization of "mediocre" or "undesirable" individuals legal.[45]

Endorsed by state Representative Harry C. Sharp, Indiana's bill was the first to legalize sterilization in a US state. Woodrow and Laughlin created a precedent of making sterilization a national priority to protect the progress of humanity by terminating "mongrel races." Indiana's law set the precedence of sterilization which became a national legal practice through the *Buck vs. Bell* case.

Carrie Buck was a seventeen-year-old woman who gave birth to a baby girl named Vivian. Buck's daughter was left in the care of her foster parents, John and Alice Dobbs. Buck was characterized as feebleminded and was sent to the Lynchburg State Colony for Epileptics and Feebleminded. Buck's mother Emma was sent there in 1920. Dr. Albert Priddy was the superintendent of the Lynchburg State Colony. Priddy was a believer in sterilization of eugenically inferior people. He performed nearly a hundred sterilizations of Virginian women in the 1910s.[46] Priddy lobbied lawmakers of the Virginia state legislature and worked with endorser of the bill Aubrey Strode to pass the Eugenical Sterilization Act of 1924, which established the Lynchburg State Colony. Unsurprisingly, he wanted to sterilize Buck as a moral delinquent and feebleminded (who was believed to have the constitution of a nine-year-old) under the new state law.

In the case *Buck vs Priddy*, Priddy rationalized that sterilization would save Virginia money and would prevent Buck from future pregnancies. Laughlin's testimony was key in the law's approval. He testified:

> All this is a typical picture of a low grade moron… The family history record and the individual case histories, if true, demonstrate the hereditary nature of the feeblemindedness and moral delinquency described in Carrie Buck. She is therefore a potential parent of socially inadequate or defective offspring.[47]

In 1924, the sterilization law was approved by the Virginia Supreme Court of Appeals, but was appealed by Irving Whitehead (Buck's attorney). The original decision was upheld and went to the US Supreme Court in October 1926. Due to Priddy's untimely death in 1925, the case was changed to *Buck vs. Bell* in 1927 because Dr. J. H. Bell was Priddy's successor and the current Lynchburg State Colony superintendent.[48] The ruling stated Buck had due process of the law and equal protection under the law in an 8 to 1 decision. The ruling upheld eugenic laws passed by other states. Buck vs. Bell set the precedent of legal sterilization on a national platform, which enforced eugenic sterilization as a social therapeutic intervention to remove less desired groups.

Prior to World War I (WWI), African Americans were ironically spared from sterilization because of segregation. However, the threat of lynching was still a reality. African Americans were not granted access to institutions that performed sterilization. That quickly changed after World War II (WWII). Post WWII, African Americans became a target of the eugenic sterilization agenda. Sterilization was a form of race-specific therapeutic intervention to "cure" American society of inferior groups who were a public health risk. This eugenic view was heightened through the passing of welfare laws in the 1930s.

Unemployment was a significant problem of the 1930s with 28% of households lacking employment.[49] Welfare and charity dependency dramatically increased, which led to the augmentation of pauperism. The results of unemployment created a eugenic epidemic with hordes of welfare dependents threatening the "genetically fit" of society. African Americans were the biggest group made dependent on welfare by the unemployment hike. Welfare dependents became a public health crisis. In 1943, Lobbyist quickly formed the Sterilization League of New Jersey, which changed to Birthright Inc. Birthright evolved from Gosney's Human Betterment Foundation into the Human Betterment Association of America (HBAA). HBAA was the only national organization sponsoring sterilization.[50] After 1950, HBAA changed their agenda from coerced sterilization to voluntary sterilization. In 1962, HBAA became Human Betterment Association for Voluntary Sterilization and made its final name change in 1965 as the Association of Voluntary Sterilization (AVS).

African Americans with and without SCA were viewed as a social disease that should be prevented from procreating and should be eradicated from society. Welfare was used to justify sterilization of Blacks who were viewed as lazy, dirty, and diseased ridden. Such perceptions encouraged the creation of ghettos. Ghettoization is to put a specific group or groups in an isolated or segregated area. There was a fear that inferior groups can cause or carry diseases, that were thought to produce an epidemic threat to the eugenically superior of society. AVS linked sterilization with welfare. AVS' president H. Curtis Wood Jr. stated that people on welfare were, "the cancer cells growing in an uncontrolled and destructive manner."[51] Furthermore, Wood asserted that welfare programs exacerbated poverty and threatened the well-being of society. The first step in preventing African Americans from overpopulating and "infecting" society was to limit procreation.

Eugenics notions influenced paranoia of African American reproduction starting in the early twentieth century. For example, the presiding justice of the *Buck vs. Bell* case, Justice Oliver Wendell Holmes Jr. stated, "Three generations of imbeciles are enough."[52] Emma, Carrie, and Vivian were viewed as feebleminded individuals and were used as an example to promote the idea that feeblemindedness was passed down generationally. The US Supreme Court felt that feeblemindedness was linked to promiscuity.[53] These ideologies were solely eugenic and the negative traits were attributed to African Americans. African American sexuality was viewed as a threat that would replenish feeblemindedness and compromise the procreative progression of an eugenically fit American society.

Chicago College of Physicians and Surgeons' Professor of Genito-Urinary Surgery and Syphilology, G. Frank Lydston was questioned about the sexual promiscuity and perversion of blacks by the American Medical Association president Hunter McGuire. McGuire wanted a scientific explanation of African Americans' perceived extreme sexual perversions. Lydston concluded, "Negro compares quite favorably as regards sexual impulses- taking all abnormalities into consideration- with the white race."[54] He believed African American sexuality was not the issue. Lydston's sexual views of African Americans were rare in his time. African American sexuality was generally perceived as insatiable and animalistic—a view associated most often with black men. Thus, the only solution for stopping the spread of criminality and the deterioration of society by African Americans and those with SCA was through castration.

Lydston was not concerned with the sexuality of African Americans, but with the eugenic threat they created through procreation. His *The Diseases of Society* advanced castration as a form of punishment and population control. "Therapeutics of Social Disease" chapter focused on solutions of criminology by two methods: controlling heredity through marriage selection and legislating sterilization to improve environments. In "The Medical Aspects of Crime," castration was used as, "a possible and permissible mode of preventing the propagation of a degenerate class of imbeciles or paupers."[55] Simultaneously, castration was used as a form of punishment in rape cases and a means of aggressive population control to stop eugenically labeled inferior groups from procreating. Castration was one form of eugenic population control. Another form was birth control.

Birth Control

Birth Control was developed and promoted by the founder of Planned Parenthood movement Margaret Sanger. Sanger was an avid eugenicist who stressed that those who are "genetically fit" should procreate and those who are "feebleminded" and "mongrels" should be prevented from reproducing. She believed birth control and eugenics are connected ideas that cannot be separated. Her speech called "Plan for Peace" in the April 1923 publication *Birth Control Review* she wanted:

> To apply a stern and rigid policy of sterilization and segregation to that grade of population whose progeny is already tainted or whose inheritance is such that objectionable traits may be transmitted to offspring and to give certain dysgenic groups in our population their choice of segregation or sterilization.[56]

Sanger along with other movers and shakers of the birth control movement, like Victoria Woodhull, Marie Stopes, Robert Dickinson, Lois Gosney-Castle, Paul Popenoe and Alan F. Guttmacher, influenced race-specific therapeutics through the eugenic practice of sterilization. The second form of eugenic population control targeted race relations and the institution of marriage.

Marriage Control

The Virginia Racial Integrity Act of 1924, influenced by the "One Drop Rule," was the "first miscegenation law in the nation passed on a eugenic basis."[57] The law made lying about one's race in registry a felony with a punishment of one to five years in prison. The eugenic social policy regarding marriage responded to the threat of miscegenation (the interbreeding of different races) within marriage. Miscegenation became a national public health crisis because the transmission of blackness by African Americans and those with SCA and other diseases endangered the purity of the white race.

The Virginia law set a national precedent which influenced numerous states. Miscegenation paranoia was a national scare tactic that influenced immigration policies to take a eugenic turn. In a eugenic mindset, not only were producing and marrying genetically inferior individuals causes of social decay, but allowing inferior groups to migrate posed another threat to the American negative eugenic agenda.

The factor of race in American immigration policy is not exclusive to the eugenic period. In 1790, President George Washington signed the Naturalization Act which asserted only "white" individuals can become citizens. In addition, the US Congress passed the first major federal immigration law restricting entry in the United States called the Chinese Exclusion Act of 1882. The Chinese Exclusion Act set the tone about race and ethnicity in twentieth century immigration policy. Eugenicists believed that immigrant entry should be no later than 1890 because most populations would be genetically undesirable.[58]

Immigrants marrying and procreating were eugenically perceived as reversing the country's progress. Laughlin had been working on immigration policy since 1920 with the US Congress and was a major influence in providing testimony and research for an immigration law to pass. Throughout the process of drafting immigration legislation, race-based pathology and eugenics influenced the proposed immigration law's terminology. In 1924, the Johnson-Reed Immigration Act passed which provided a national origins quota system allowing two percent of the nationality's population, with Asia being completely excluded. The

Act was purposefully enforced to prevent individuals characterized as black from entering the county due to fear of spreading SCA.

Linus Pauling

Sterilization through population control, marriage control, and immigration shaped African Americans' and SCA carriers' illness and identity. The results were scientific theorizing, clinical discovery, and political transformation. SCA became significant in the 1950s and 1960s because it served as the archetype that influenced the relevancy of molecular biology through post WWII medicine. Molecular biology of the mid-twentieth century was the equivalent and foundation of the Human Genome Project in the late twentieth century. The key player in molecular biology was Linus Pauling.

In 1948, the California Institute of Technology pioneered in the method of electrophoresis. Electrophoresis is the separation of molecules according to their electrical charge, which determined the difference between normal and sickled hemoglobin.[59] In 1949, the California Institute of Technology's Chemist, Linus Pauling published an article in the *Science* journal entitled "Sickle-Cell Anemia, A Molecular Disease," which explained individuals that carried SCA had a different electric charge compared to individuals who did not carry the disease. In the same year, SCA was named the first molecular disease by Pauling. This was significant because it leads to the hypothesis that the cause of SCA may be an altered molecular structure, and genes determined the precise structure of proteins.

Pauling classified SCA as a "black-race disorder" and suggested sickle cell was the consequence of a molecular mutation in the hemoglobin. As a result, Pauling inadvertently discovered RBM. In contrast, Emmel's test identified the characteristics of SCA. Pauling's discovery transformed the understanding of SCA, and took the understanding of disease in general to another level. The concepts of racial purity and disease were prevalent among American scientists who declared, "Sickle cell anemia in American blacks (who by definition, it was assumed, had white ancestry) was a perfect example of how race mixture can be disadvantageous in its racial effects."[60] Once again, SCA went from a proxy for race to a consequence of race.

Pauling and his scientists concluded sickle cell affected black Americans (hybrids) more than Africans (pure) who possessed the sickle cell trait. As a result of this conclusion, theories of racial admixture (the mixing of races through marriage, sex, and cohabitation) developed and advanced the idea that race can affect disease risk and severity. Pauling's finding earned him a Nobel Prize in Chemistry in 1954.[61] Pauling's influence on race, research, and medicine is reflected in the creation of the first race-based drug BiDil, which I will discuss in chapter three. SCA was not the only inherited disease that had systemic racial influence in the late nineteenth and twentieth centuries. Eugenic influences affected TSD and the Jewish population.

Tay Sachs Disease

Tay Sachs Disease (gangliosidoses or cerebral sphingolipidoses) is a rare inherited disorder that progressively destroys nerve cells (neurons) in the brain and spinal cord. TSD is a mutation affecting the development of the "Hex A" enzyme. The "Hex A" enzyme has an important function that controls the amount of fat in the nervous system and the brain. When the enzyme is not working properly, excess fat accumulates resulting in neurological deterioration. Tay-Sachs is one of the most severe of childhood disorders. TSD symptoms include hyperacusis (decreased sound tolerance or "DST"), social withdrawal, mental retardation, cherry-red spots on the retinas, enlargement of the head due to the increase of water around the brain, and alteration in muscle tone. Eventually, the child becomes immobile, visually impaired, and dies by age four.[62] Similar to SCA, a person inherits TSD through Mendelian markers of abnormal/recessive genes—one from each parent.

In 1881, TSD was first described by British Opthalmologist and surgeon Warren Tay. Tay's observation of TSD led the British Opthalmalogical Society to publish its first volume. After Tay's first observation, he stated,

Mrs. L. brought her infant, 12 months of age, to see Tay at his office in London on March 7, 1881 "in the hope that something might be done to strengthen it" (1881:55). This baby was unable to hold "its" head up or move its limbs, and when asked about the baby's eyesight, the mother replied "she did not think her baby took as much notice as other babies.[63]

Tay's visual observations developed the precedent on TSD symptoms, with Bernard Sachs to follow.

In 1887, Jewish Neurologist Bernard Sachs was one of America's premier clinical neurologists. His first experience of TSD was when he saw brownish/cherry red spots in a two-year-old girl's eyes. He classified TSD as "Amaurotic Family Idiocy"[64] a mental and optical condition that was a hereditary trait. Sachs concluded,

Taking all these histories into account as they have been reported by a number of different observers, there can be no doubt that the cases described by the oculists [ophthalmologists] are identical with those seen by me, and they constitute a very definite family affection due to the occurrence of the affection in several members of the same family.[65]

The disease ultimately was referred to as Tay Sachs, named after Warren Tay, and Bernard Sachs the discoverers of the disease. The validation of TSD's hereditary status made Jews vulnerable to the eugenic idea that race was a marker of disease.

TSD was generalized as a Jewish disease. In 1894, Dr. Curtis B. Carter labeled TSD as "a disease among the Hebrews" and in 1895 Sachs told the New York Neurological Society that TSD was a disease "almost exclusively Jewish."[66] TSD was primarily from the Ashkenazis Jews from Eastern Europe—a development discovered in the 1930s. TSD was categorized as belonging to a sub group within the Jewish population. In contrast, SCA was generalized as a black disease, not considering the numerous backgrounds from which those considered Black came. However, that did not stop the association of Jewishness and TSD. Before the turn of the twentieth century, eugenic bias purported that TSD was a contagious disease, causing fear of pandemic.

For example, Neurologist Dr. Isador H. Coriat alleged in one of his cases that TSD nerve cells contained poison that was transmitted through Jewish mother's milk.[67]

Furthermore, the danger of a Jewish mother breastfeeding was emphasized by Neurologist William Hirsch. In 1898, Hirsch observed a case in which he asserted many children became infected with TSD by the same mother, which "obviously" explained why the family suffered from TSD. Hirsch encouraged stopping the practice of breast feeding, suggesting, "That as soon as the diagnosis of such a case has been made, the child be taken from its mother's breast, and all future children be fed with other nourishment."[68] Jewish breastfeeding was perceived to be a means of degeneration that threatened the well-being of the defined "genetically fit" society.

TSD, a mental and nervous disease, was categorized as a form of fee-blemindedness. Goddard, through the Binet-Simon intelligence tests, found that 60% of Jews were classified as morons.[69] The test consisted of various pictures and was meant for immigrants who did not speak English. The hierarchy of intelligence started with the "Nordic stocks" of Canadians, Scandinavians, British, Scottish, and Dutch. The lower stocks of intelligence were Jews, Polish (Poles), and Greeks with the Negro as the least intelligent. Princeton Psychologist Carl C. Brigham asserted, "The intellectual superiority of our Nordic group over Alpine, Mediterranean and Negro groups."[70] Goddard and many eugenicists' views on Jews and other races were influenced by a philosophical giant Immanuel Kant.

Kant viewed Jews (and other races like Blacks) as lesser human beings, and described Judaism as a superstitious, dishonest, and a materialistic religion. In 2003, the United Jewish Appeal of Toronto states,

> Going back to at least the twelfth century, European culture had developed a rich and ghastly tableau of imaginary Jews... Kant's division of humanity reiterated and reinvigorated the religious and racial hierarchies of the past... He took this earlier religious hostility toward Jews and reformulated it in philosophical language... Kant set the stage for modern secular anti-Semitism... [and] provided the framework for future anti-Semites.[71]

Eugenic and Kantian influences inflamed the perception of Jews as inferior. TSD classified Jewish people, whether they had the disease or not, as social outcasts. Russian Zionist Max Mandelstamm stated that Jews were a degenerate people, "that the decrepit, miserable, weak bodily constitution of the Jews of the ghetto is the exclusive result of their wretched social and economic situation."[72] Similar to African Americans, Jews were viewed as disease-ridden people susceptible to numerous kinds of illnesses. Jewish women were affected more by female-related diseases than women in other races. Negative TSD and other pathological connotations toward Jews created stigmas like the 'nervous" or "insane" Jew. Eugenic ideologies placed Jews within the social agendas of marriage, reproduction, and immigration policies tailored as race-specific cures of the Jewish problem.

Intermarriage Control

Eugenics influenced the father of Zionist Movement and social scientist Arthur Ruppin. Zionism was a political movement aimed at creating a Jewish homeland in Israel. He believed Jewish intermarriage produced negative racial consequences. Ruppin's proposed nation state would not be based on religion, but rather ethnic and national identity. Ruppin believed intermarriage would dramatically alter the physical, cultural and spiritual distinctions of Jewishness. In the 1904 publication *The Jews of Today* publishing, Ruppin stated Jews,

> Whose facial physiognomy displays none of the traits of the so-called Jewish type, whose morphological type cannot be identified as of Jewish descent is substantial. Therewith the last bridge, racial unity, connecting eastern and western Jewry, divided as they are already culturally, will be destroyed. And since their bond with eastern European Jewry has vanished and they stand alone, the absorption of western European Jewry will happen quite easily.[73]

Ruppin's idea of intermarriage created an interesting binary. First, intermarriage was disliked from a Jewish Zionist perspective because it threatened one's identity. Second, intermarriage was disliked from an American eugenic perspective because TSD compromised the eugenic ideal of racial purity. Both concepts embraced and justified racial identity and exclusivism. Ruppin viewed intermarriage as a schism that would cause the fragmentation of Judaism.

America's framework has always produced a heterogeneous society. Eugenics promoted an "us and them" narcissistic mentality of constructed racial pride. An important aspect of racial pride was the concept of reproduction, which brought hope for a socially fit future. Since TSD was a children's disease, the fear of a generation gap and social inadequacy intensified. Eugenicist and professor of Neurology at Tufts College Medical School Abraham Myerson believed insanity and feeblemindedness were traits of TSD. In his 1925 book The Inheritance of Mental Diseases, Myerson suggested that epilepsy has many pathological origins in its nature. In 1933, Davenport's newspaper *Eugenical News* commended Germany on their eugenics movement, which included eugenic journals like the *Archiv für Rassen- und Gesellschaftsbiologie* (Archive for Race and Society Biology).[74] In 1936, Germany awarded Laughlin an honorary Doctor of Medicine.

In 1935, in the Archives of Neurology and Psychiatry, Myerson published "A Critique of Proposed 'Ideal' Sterilization Legislation." He powerfully argued against mass sterilization, but hypocritically justified the sterilization of Communists, Capitalists, and Jews. *Buck vs. Bell* was indirectly used by Myerson to justify abortions of Jewish babies due to TSD. Myerson felt Jews were, "those restless and reckless persons who fail because they attempt too much, but who care the ferment by which the mass is lifted."[75] Myerson's "mass" was the burden of perceived inferior individuals like the Jews. Hindering reproduction was the solution to prevent the spread of TSD. At the time, the eugenic use of intermarriage and reproductive restrictions supposedly protected the social elect. However, the most influential policy to prevent the "infiltration" of Jews to America was immigration restriction.

Immigration

The Industrial Revolution created menial and unskilled jobs which were often filled by immigrants. The Jews "not-quite-white" status was connected to the presence of Jewish immigrants in such jobs. Racial biology created classifications that formed social boundaries and segregated American citizens. Jews (as well as Irish, Polish, and Italians) were the different type of whites, the mining and manufacturing workers socially placed in the lower class while making white owners of industrial empires wealthy.[76] The classism of labor classified industrial owners as the "genetically fit" and the labor workers as the "unfit," connecting business practice with Darwinism. Whiteness was not solely skin deep, but reflected economics, power, political and social means starting from the middle class; an idea that hindered Jews from claiming the classification and attribution of "Whiteness" until mid-twentieth century.

Immigrants were often viewed as the enemy, blamed for deflating wages, accused of abusing public assistance, and considered a public health threat. For example, in 1892, typhus and cholera infected New York City. New immigrants were detained and placed in a quarantine station off Staten Island.[77] Nationalism (citizens identifying with one's nation) was replaced by nativism (protecting the interests of native-born or established inhabitants against immigrants). Being an American took on a different meaning, depending on who you were. The American "melting pot metaphor" promoting diversity and unity was a far cry from eugenic ideology. Only certain groups were accepted into the melting pot. Other groups like African Americans and Jews were considered the fire to help heat the pot, or even the spoon to help stir the pot, but by no means the movers and shakers of America.

Jews left Eastern Europe to start a new life free from the anti-Semitism that led to persecution and eventually genocide. Unfortunately, Jews did not escape the social constructions that questioned their humanity and worth. American society viewed Jews as an inbreeding and racially incestuous type of people; qualities not viewed as American. In immigration conversations, eugenic thought used TSD as a proxy for racial ideological purposes, much like SCA that was associated with African Americans. Eugenic ideology vehemently asserted that Jewish assimilation into American society did not improve social and public health. Viennese physician Martin Englander endorsed the link between Jewish assimilation and degeneration. He stated, "The startling frequency of illness among the Jewish race."[78] Englander claimed in his 1902 study that there was a statistical connection between middle-class western European Jews and higher rates of alcoholism, mental and nervous disorders, and suicide. Physician Hugo Hoppe cited statistics similar to Englander's with criminality as a trait among assimilated Jews.

The Jewish "parasite" and "germ" were powerful anti-Semitic images and designations that permeated within the American perception of Jews. Negative racial Jewish perceptions, Alan Kraut states,

> sought to sketch the Jew as a public health menace, one who might end up on the public relief roles in droves, deficient in the physical vitality to stand the test of the rugged American environment, as did the pioneer forbearers of the native-born and the sturdier stock that had emigrated to the United States from Northern and Western Europe.[79]

Whereas African Americans were viewed as brutish and primal, Jews were viewed as fickle individuals who could not physically handle the burden of assimilation. US Navy Medical Director Dr. Manly H. Simons acknowledged immigrant Jews,' "increasing degradation, retardation, and extinction to an inability to adapt their genetic constitution to their new circumstances."[80] Simons, influenced by the Mendelian technique, noted family disease like TSD lead to early death or sterility. These assumptions were based on alleged and repeated hereditary racial qualities in Jews.

There was a continued fear that degeneration would wipe out white American civilization. Racial and medical discourse of TSD and SCA were bound with ideological views on immigration and race. Doctors and other medical professionals became instigators who ingrained their research, study, and medical voice with eugenic and nativist discourse. These individuals became medical antagonists, taking an issue that was mainly social presenting it as a biological one that threatened the well-being of American society. Hence, immigration was a race-specific cure or a "social antibiotic" that would lessen the diseased Jewish presence in America.

Officer of the American Eugenics Society and Vice President of the Immigration Restriction League, Madison Grant asserted that immigration would degrade America's Nordic racial constitution. He believed, "the man of old stock is being crowded out of many country districts by these foreigners just as he is to-day being literally driven off the streets of New York City by the swarms of Polish Jews."[81] New York University Professor of Sociology Henry Pratt Fairchild asserted that TSD met the definition of an "Excludable Medical Condition" described in the 1903 *Book of Instructions for the Medical Inspection of Immigrants*, which indicated that mental defectiveness, among other conditions, was "excluded by the immigration law."[82]

The same ideology was embraced by German-Jewish anthropologist Franz Boas. Boas primary research was on the anatomy of Jewish immigrants. His earliest studies were the head forms of Jews. Boas studies were an assimilationist example of physical anthropology, which had a major influence on immigration policy. In the 1903 journal *American Anthropologist*, he published "Heredity in Headform." The article examined the relationship between inheritance and head forms comparing it to Mendel's research and hypothesis. Boas' article had case studies of forty-nine Jewish families organized by Maurice Fishberg.

Maurice Fishberg was a New York physician and anthropologist, and his research had profound influence on Boas. For example, Boas' article on "Race, Immigration, and Assimilation, Changes in Bodily Form of Descendants of Immigrants," was heavily influenced by Fishberg's studies. Boas article was a key source in the 1911 forty volume study of the U.S. Congress Immigration policy. The study "symbolized the high point of political propaganda for immigration restriction before the immigration laws were enacted in the twenties. The investigation should be directed towards an inquiry into 1) the assimilation or stability of type, and 2) changes in the characteristics of the development of the individual."[83]

TSD cases reported prior to the 1924 Johnson-Reed Immigration Act contained racist and nativist language, associating Jews with nervous diseases like TSD due to their racial inferiority. From 1913 to 1918, Physician Isador Coriat asserted, "[e]ven if the parents are apparently healthy, they have probably inherited a nervous disposition from their persecuted and maltreated ancestors. The Jew possesses certain racial characteristics of organic inferiority through which he differs from the non- Jew."[84]

The 1924 Johnson-Reed Immigration Act was influenced by eugenicists like Fishberg, Boas, and Laughlin. The only way to prevent integration was to frame a structure of encapsulation among Jews, which the ghetto concept was used as a solution. Homogeneous neighborhoods were a eugenic justification for racist and biased real estate and mortgage practices. The premise was that immigration could not keep every undesirable group of people out of the country. The idea of putting the same "type" of people in a specific location to maintain homogeneity; such action would prevent intermarriage, reproductive issues and protect the socially fit. Such ideologies continued well into the twentieth century through the passing of the GI Bill, which limited blacks and Latinos to the rental housing market and excluded access to home ownership. Advocacy against racist real estate practices resulted in the passing of the Fair Housing Act of 1968. However, race continued to be influential in real estate well into the twenty first century.

The Eugenics Movement influenced race-based social policies, which were viewed as therapeutic interventions or cures to prevent an American infection by undesirable groups, including African Americans and Jews with and without SCA and TSD. The classifications of SCA as "a black disease" and TSD as "a Jewish disease" constructed false perceptions of tailored research and technology for specific racial groups, which made race a proxy in medicine. In chapter two, I will examine misunderstandings, perceptions, experimentation, consequences, and African Americans' response relating to the RBM and the black body.

Notes

1. SCA and TSD are diseases that are prevalent in numerous racial groups. They are not homogeneic diseases. I will expound more on SCA and TSD and their relation to racial groups later in this chapter.
2. Stern, *Eugenic Nation*, 14.
3. Bethencourt, Francisco. *Racisms: From the Crusades to the Twentieth Century*. Princeton University Press, 2014, 276–288.

4. Sussman, *The Myth of Race*, 48.
5. Ibid.
6. Ibid., 49.
7. Stern, *Eugenic Nation*, 11.
8. Hansen, Randall, and Desmond S. King. *Sterilized by the State: Eugenics, Race, and the Population Scare in Twentieth-Century North America*. New York: Cambridge University Press, 2013, 29.
9. Ibid.
10. Ibid., 32.
11. Hansen and King, *Sterilized by the State*, 32.
12. Sussman, *The Myth of Race*, 51.
13. Sussman, *The Myth of Race*, 50.
14. Hansen and King, *Sterilized by the State*, 33.
15. Ibid., 34.
16. Ibid.
17. Stern, *Eugenic Nation*, 11.
18. Sussman, *The Myth of Race*, 55.
19. Hansen and King, *Sterilized by the State*, 37–47.
20. Ibid., 57.
21. Ibid., 56.
22. Largent, *Breeding Contempt*, 47.
23. Ibid., 48.
24. McBride, *From TB to AIDS*, 19–20.
25. Ibid., 48.
26. Sussman, *The Myth of Race*, 70.
27. Wailoo, Keith. *Dying in the City of the Blues: Sickle Cell Anemia and the Politics of Race and Health*. Chapel Hill: University of North Carolina Press, 2001, 55.
28. Ibid., 5.
29. Savitt, Todd Lee. *Race and Medicine in Nineteenth- and Early-Twentieth-Century America*. Kent, OH: Kent State University Press, 2007, 18.
30. Ibid., 25.
31. McBride, *From TB to AIDS*, 16.
32. Ibid., 50.
33. McBride, *From TB to AIDS*, 17.
34. Ibid., 58–63.
35. Balgir, R. S. "Indigenous and Independent Origin of the B*-Mutation in Ancient India: Is It a Myth or Reality?" *Mankind Quarterly* 42, no. 2 (Winter 2001), 108–109.

36. Wailoo, *Drawing Blood*, 142.
37. Savitt, *Race and Medicine*, 42.
38. Savitt, *Race and Medicine*, 42.
39. Tapper, Melbourne. *In the Blood: Sickle Cell Anemia and the Politics of Race*. Philadelphia: University of Pennsylvania Press, 1999, 16.
40. Wailoo, *Drawing Blood*, 150.
41. Wailoo, *Dying in the City of the Blues*, 89.
42. McBride, *From TB to AIDS*, 138.
43. Pollock, Anne. *Medicating Race: Heart Disease and Durable Preoccupations with Difference*. Durham: Duke University Press, 2012, 40.
44. Largent, *Breeding Contempt*, 66.
45. Sussman, *The Myth of Race*, 54.
46. Hansen and King, *Sterilized by the State*, 104.
47. Largent, *Breeding Contempt*, 100.
48. Hansen and King, *Sterilized by the State*, 105.
49. Hansen and King, *Sterilized by the State*, 238.
50. Ibid., 238–239.
51. Hansen and King, *Sterilized by the State*, 239.
52. Largent, *Breeding Contempt*, 102.
53. Ibid., 101.
54. Largent, *Breeding Contempt*, 25–26.
55. Ibid., 27.
56. Schrag, Peter. *Not Fit for Our Society: Nativism and Immigration*. Berkeley: University of California Press, 2010, 94.
57. Largent, *Breeding Contempt*, 65.
58. Sussman, *The Myth of Race*, 100.
59. Pauling, Linus, et al. *Linus Pauling: Scientist and Peacemaker*. Corvallis: Oregon State University Press, 2001, 129.
60. Fullwiley, Duana. "The Biologistical Construction of Race: 'Admixture' Technology and the New Genetic Medicine." *Social Studies of Science* 38, no. 5 (October 2008), 695 (Sage Publications Ltd.).
61. Pauling et al., *Linus Pauling*, 133.
62. Reuter, "The Genuine Jewish," 296.
63. Ibid., 297.
64. Reuter, "The Genuine Jewish," 297.
65. Ibid.
66. Ibid., 299.
67. Ibid., 298.
68. Reuter, "The Genuine Jewish," 298.

69. Schrag, *Not Fit for Our Society*, 8.
70. Ibid.
71. Sussman, *The Myth of Race*, 29.
72. Hart, Mitchell B. "Articles—Racial Science, Social Science, and the Politics of Jewish Assimilation." *Isis* 90, no. 2 (1999), 276.
73. Hart, "Racial Science," 278.
74. Washington, *Medical Apartheid*, 193–194.
75. Largent, *Breeding Contempt*, 99.
76. Brodkin, Karen. *How Jews Became White Folks and What That Says About Race in America*. New Brunswick, NJ: Rutgers University Press, 1998, 55.
77. Reuter, "The Genuine Jewish Type," 306.
78. Hart, "Racial Science," 278.
79. Ibid., 285.
80. Reuter, "The Genuine Jewish Type," 308.
81. Ibid.
82. Reuter, "The Genuine Jewish Type," 309.
83. Hart, "Racial Science," 287.
84. Reuter, "The Genuine Jewish Type," 310.

3

Maleficence Toward the Minority Patient

The idea of race-based medicine creates maleficence (harm) in minority patient care. Eugenic influence created false assumptions and stereotypes (the homogeneity of characteristics, experience, and behavior of a group and individuals from that group) about the black patient's body. Physicians' infatuation of the black body created a disturbing language, which caused unconscionable harm in the clinical practice. Inaccurate semantics and perceptions provided the justification for inhumane experimentation on black bodies. Racial history speaks to the eerie ideological weight of race and biology, illustrating how racial stereotypes disrupt clinical judgment and induce implicit bias. As a result, deeply rooted mistrust remains at the core of African Americans and their participation in the clinical process. This chapter will examine the maleficence of minority patients through misappropriations of the black body, race-based experimentation, consequences of such misappropriations, and African Americans' response to race-based experimentation.

© The Author(s) 2019
K. A. Johnson, *Medical Stigmata*,
https://doi.org/10.1007/978-981-13-2992-0_3

Misappropriations of the Black Body

As discussed in Chapter 1, the historical usage of race in medicine and research has undermined the human worth of communities of color and led to genetic and biological propaganda. For over 400 years, the human development of the concept of race has not promoted ethical engagement, solidarity, and literacy but has instead been used to oppress, exclude, and dehumanize individuals and groups. Human history has demonstrated the use of race has replaced prudence and practical wisdom with antagonistic and apathetic treatment toward black human beings. Consider, for example, the physical stereotypes of African Americans.

The eugenic perceptions of the "black body" produced misappropriations and falsified theories of the anatomy and biology of black individuals. Darwinism and human variation studies were used to form ideologies that viewed black individuals as subhuman, with physiological attributes like apes.[1] It also justified the concept of racial hierarchy—that is, the assertion that one's own race is superior to other races. Such beliefs challenged the personhood of African Americans.

Personhood

The era of slavery and the eugenics movement both altered the personhood of African Americans. The auction block of slavery made black bodies a public spectacle with law and medicine defining the black body's worth and aesthetics. The stain of anti-black body discourse remained in American society. African Americans had the unique experience of surrogacy, having their private faculties of their bodies, but no bodily ownership.

This oddity of bodily experience was evident not only in the institution of slavery, but also in the terrorism of lynching in the late nineteenth century and mid-twentieth century, the Jim Crow era's separate but equal legal status, punishment for challenging the status quo in the Civil Rights era, and excessive physical force between the police and communities of color. The physical degradation and death of black bodies rarely if ever receive justice or accountability. One reason is the notion of privacy. As Dr. Karla F. C. Halloway suggests, "Privacy is presumed to be a fundamental right of personhood."[2] Privacy and vulnerability are linked together. If you can take away someone's privacy and vulnerability, you can take away their personhood. Citizenship grants privacy along with status, rights, privileges, and responsibilities that are withheld from a non-citizen. Thus, American history made black bodies private entities in public discourse.[3] As a consequence, black bodies' value, identity, and autonomy were compromised by law and medicine.

Autonomy, in the Greek, means *autos* (self) *nomos* (rule, governance, or law).[4] Individual autonomy is free of controlling agents and limitations. Autonomy gives one the freedom and the capacity to have self-rule and perform intentional actions. Autonomy is important because what controls a person controls their destiny. If one cannot control their own destiny, that individual is simply a pawn with no liberty to adequately thrive and express oneself. Liberty and agency are the principals of personhood; without them no individual can attain their full potential. As Dr. Holloway mentions,

> A critical distinction lies in what Rubenfeld explains as the juxtaposition of a (human) person's claim to self-identity and the (social) person's acknowledgment of the interior (private) and exterior (public) locations of self. Liberty cannot be a claim of individuality when individual identity is filtered through our associations or assignments to identity categories. Similarly, mirroring the way that an individual cannot liberate herself from the communitarian claims of social personhood, social, political and legal citizenships have assigned a differential ethical value to particular kinds of citizens at different moments in our history.[5]

An individual or a group with assigned identities and diminished autonomy, controlled by social systems, laws, and those of influence, cannot adequately act on their desires and plans.

The black body's autonomy has been compromised by its regulation, surveillance, and misappropriation. Western society, rooted in xenophobic systems, perpetuates a systemic discourse regarding the inferiority of black bodies meant to keep such individuals "in their place" and hinder any kind of autonomous action. Black bodies are disrespected because of Western ideas, actions, and attitudes that "ignore, insult, demean, or are inattentive to others' rights of autonomous action."[6] As a result, black bodies have never been valued and respected, which sustains challenges of self-worth and self-esteem that continue to exist in the black community.

The inconsideration of the black body's autonomy jeopardizes the other three fundamental principles of biomedical ethics: non-maleficence (doing no harm), beneficence (doing good), and justice (what is deserved). When the black body's autonomy is devalued non-maleficence, beneficence, and justice cannot be accomplished. Furthermore, the black body being hindered from autonomy leaves it in a dependent discourse of stereotypes and preconceptions that takes away self-identification.[7] The ideologies of African Americans being "lesser than" or "inferior" transferred into the fields of anthropology, anatomy, and biology, creating myths of innate human differences.

Pseudo-Biology

American medicine and research influenced the perverse overreaction to African Americans' physiological and anatomical traits which produced unsettling claims that portray blacks as extra-terrestrial beings. In categorical order, the black body was viewed as abnormal. The physiological misappropriations of blacks were judgements comparing visual biological differences between blacks and whites.

A well-known racist southern physician, Samuel Cartwright, was influential assigning alien attributions to the black body. He asserted the black body was different than the white body in every way. Cartwright said,

> It is not only in the skin that a difference of color exists between the negro and the white man, but in the membranes, the muscles, the tendons, and in all the fluids and secretions. Even the negro brain and nerves, the chyle and all the humors, are tintured with a shade of the pervading darkness. His bile is of a deeper color, and his blood is blacker than the white man's.[8]

Every physician did not agree with Cartwright's ideas of the black body, but such ideas fueled racist perceptions of blacks. The pseudo-biological addiction of the black body created systemic descriptions that led to myths of black people's physiques.

The belief that black bodies were innately different produced the terms "black hardiness" and "black durability." These are the notions that African Americans have the innate capacity to endure or tolerate extreme conditions or illnesses. It was thought that the experience of slavery made African Americans evolve into a people of great endurance and stamina. Such ideas were used as an explanation of how blacks survived the sin of slavery. The understanding was the black body had to be abnormal because the humanity of a white body did not have the capacity to endure what black bodies experienced. Cartwright associated black hardiness with the physiognomy of blacks. Cartwright stated, "Black skin, thick lips, flat nose- corresponded to an intensification of vitality and physical strength."[9] It was also believed that African Americans did not get eating disorders due to their "gastric hardiness."[10] The durability of the skull and skeleton of blacks were popular tropes among anthropologists.

The skulls of African Americans were deemed to be smaller than whites, implying that the "black brain" was not as developed as whites. As a result, blacks could not reach the same intellectual capacity of whites. Furthermore, black people skulls were thought to rapidly thicken at puberty, and thus "the animal portion of the brain then became supreme, ruling over the adult Negro organism."[11] The "animal portion" of the African Americans brain allegedly hindered social mobility, intellectual and social progress. Therefore, blacks were stuck in the same primitive state since their inception.

In 1859, German anthropologist Theodor Waitz said that one use of thick black skulls was is in fighting. Waitz said, "Negroes, men and women, butt each other like rams without exhibiting much sensibility."[12] Also, he believed that the black skeleton was heavier, thicker and larger than a European's. Waitz's colleague anthropologist Carl Vogt agreed that blacks use their skulls to fight like rams. In 1860, a woman novelist stated that it is physically impossible to knock a slave out down to the ground because black skulls were so thick that the skull would bruise or break the slave-owner's hand.[13] The next black features viewed differently were the eyes, ears and legs.

The eyesight and hearing of blacks were thought to be super human and extremely sensitive in various environments. Samuel Cartwright asserted, "The negro's hearing is better. His sight stronger and he seldom needs spectacles."[14] The legs of blacks were thought to be different based on the hormonal theory or gland theory of racial difference proposed by British anthropologist Arthur Keith. Keith's argued that the dissimilarities of whites and blacks were caused by the functioning of endocrine glands. Keith concluded, "The long 'storklike legs' of some Negroid types have been thought by some to be due to abeyance of interstitial gland action."[15] The glands of blacks had to be different because it explained the physical advantages blacks possessed compared to whites. Blacks' longer limbs and shorter trunks was the reason why blacks could run faster than any group. In 1964, Anthropologist J. M. Tanner continued belief that black bodies were different. He suggested that African Americans had longer arms and legs, heavier bones, narrower hips, and shorter trunks compared to whites.[16]

Even the joints, body fat, and muscle fibers of blacks were believed to have peculiarities. Blacks (particularly black athletes) were double-jointed, which allowed hyper-extensibility, an idea claimed by Anthropologist Edward E. Hunt Jr.[17] Blacks has less body fat than whites, which contributed to their physical advantage. In the 1964 Tokyo Olympics, James E. Counsilman of Indiana University believed that black athletes had more muscle fibers. Mr. Counsilman said,

> I believe that the black athlete has more white muscle fibers. Oversimplifying it, every muscle has two types of fibers – white fibers and red fibers. The white muscle fibers are adapted for speed of movement, otherwise power. The red muscle fibers are adapted for endurance... I think the difference in muscle fibers is the reason the black athlete is a better sprinter.[18]

Racial differences did not end with comparing the physiology of black and whites. The discourse continued with constructing pathological difference among races.

The *Southern Medical Journal* (*SMJ*) was a key contributor to medical myths about the black body. In 1934, *SMJ* indicates,

> Syphilis behaves differently in the white and the negro, and attacks the various organs and systems of the body with different force. One can only wonder how much of the negro's reaction to disease is different from the Caucasian because of *native endowments, structural and functional.* That the negro has *anatomical peculiarities*, is prone to certain diseases and relatively free of others is recognized. (emphasis added)[19]

It was the language of medical journals like *SMJ* that made race a proxy for pathology.

Since blacks and whites were viewed as opposite types of beings, physicians believed that black and white illnesses happened seasonally. The Association of American Anatomists was very assertive to "keep a careful record of all variations and anomalies between whites and blacks."[20] It was believed that blacks' vulnerability to become sick was in the winter and spring and whites became sick in the summer and autumn. There were even inquires if antibiotic therapy had different reactions between blacks and whites.[21] Heat was another factor that affected the illnesses of blacks and whites.

The notion of "heat tolerance" is the belief that blacks innately can endure higher temperatures than whites. This was the general view among slaveholders. Black slaves were in the heat all day without any perceived physical deterioration. Inquiries regarding whether blacks' sweat was different emerged because it had an intense smell. Cartwright believed that blacks' heat tolerance was an "ethical peculiarity in harmony with their efficiency as laborers in hot, damp, close, suffocating atmospheres- where instead of suffering and dying, as the white man would, they are healthier, happier and more prolific than in their native Africa."[22] The main trait that was believed to aid blacks in the sun was their skin.

Black skin was the essential symbol of hardiness. It was the symbol that superseded all other black characteristics that marked blacks to be inferior. Black skin was viewed as thick and tough. Its alleged thickness was "credited with an increase resistance to both infection and diseases such as scarlet fever, erysipelas, and measles."[23] Even in the late twentieth century, it was believed that black skin decreased the number and penetration of mosquito bites. The South Carolina physician, C. W. Kollock suggested,

> The black man's skin, the most obvious mark of inferiority, was believed to possess certain peculiar qualities other than distinctiveness of color. It secreted oil which kept it in a state of shine, thus deflecting intense solar rays. The pigment carried heat into the system, there driving water to the surface, which in evaporation dissipated body heat. The negro made an excellent worker because he was eminently a sweating animal; but this remarkable sweating capacity, however is useful in the field, caused him to be a pariah in white society, objectionable in the jury box, the legislature, or the drawing room. During Radical Reconstruction the 'sweetness of loyalty perfumed the air' of legislature and political meeting, and white men held their noses.[24]

As discussed, the skin and other traits of African Americans were used to sustain the black hardiness theory. The binary of super-human and sub-human applications of the black body were complex and contradictory. The hardiness of blacks can be misinterpreted as a positive trait, but such descriptions were viewed as primal and inferior. Both black hardiness and the perceived human inferiority of blacks were means to justify suffering and exploitation.

The assumed durability of blacks proved the foundation for the ideology of "the pain-resistant Negro." Blacks' thick skin and sensitive nervous system made them endure whippings without feeling pain.[25] Black women did not feel pain in child birth. African Americans were considered best in surgery, because "they are stoic in their reaction to pain and discomfiture, do not easily go into shock, take anesthesia well, resist infection, and show remarkable powers of recovery."[26] Even heart surgery and glaucoma physicians felt they did not cause African Americans pain. A 1932 and 1952 physician's report stated that two black patients, one who had surgery and another who lost eyesight, handled pain and symptoms extremely well and did not use treatment until pain was a factor.[27]

The myth of the black body and its defiance to pain created the perception that African Americans were mystical and black bodies possessed magical powers. Black skin was believed to have special healing powers, a black person's saliva cured thrush, and Appalachian folk medicine believed the spit of a very dark skinned black with "blue gums" could cure ringworm.[28] Even the lung capacity and function of black people were understood to be different, which was examined in Lundy Braun's book *Breathing Race into the Machine: The Surprising Career of the Spirometer from Plantation to Genetics*. Such ideas of black hardiness and mysticism influenced and transferred into clinical research.

Race-Based Experimentation

Race-based experimentation was the American medicine community's response to the misappropriations of the black body. Experimentation on blacks started in the slave era. Slave owners and physicians developed ideologies and procedures that set the unethical precedent of the clinical process for African Americans. Unethical treatment of blacks continued through the military, which chose blacks for harmful clinical projects. This same treatment continued within the prison systems. The "uniqueness" of the African American body constructed by racial biology justified the need for the harmful clinical experiments and led to two binaries of clinical research.

First, the black body (and that of other races) needed to be examined to understand specific racial anomalies, disorders, and illnesses. Through the sustained notion of black hardiness, the first binary sustained maleficence to black bodies and disrupted the autonomy of black patients through the physical afflictions experiments left on the body. Second, the black body was used to expand knowledge of anatomy, pathology, epidemiology, disability, and physiological reactions to certain drugs and substances.

These two binaries created as Michel Foucalt coined the "clinical gaze" or the "medical gaze." In Dr. Cynthia Davis' book *Bodily and Narrative Forms: The Influence of Medicine on American Literature*,[29] *1845–1915*, she mentions Foucalt's definition of the term,

The clinical gaze is a gaze of the concrete sensibility, a gaze that travels from body to body as a simple unconceptualized confrontation of a gaze, a face, or a glance and a silent body. The empirical and non-reciprocal nature of such confrontations depends upon the medical eye remaining both the depository and source of clarity were it would be clouded by doubt, by emotions, its clinical authority would risk being undermined, subjecting the clinician to the sort of scrutiny he sought to employ with others and avert from himself.[30]

The "looking down" and "looking over" black human beings value created the self-inverted gaze with whites being spectators and participants in clinical racial scopophilia.[31]

"Clinical Trial" is a term used in the twentieth century in the competitive area of research and science. Clinical comes from the twentieth century expansion of the word clinic with clinical meaning "coldly detached."[32] It replaced the taboo term "medical experiment." In Latin, experiment means *ex* (from or out of) and *periculum* (a dangerous trial).[33] A clinical trial can be used for therapeutic and non-therapeutic purposes. Curiosity, human detachment, combined with the black hardiness ideology, led to the desensitization about harming black bodies in American medical experimentation.[34] Such experimental processes started during the slave era.

Slave Experimentation

The areas where slaves lived on the plantation were called the slave quarters. It was in such locations where most of the clinical work on slaves were done. Slave quarters were known as "Slave Hospitals" or "Clinic Wards."[35] Since the belief of race strongly asserted biological difference, different treatment of blacks made sense because one was dealing with a different type of body and personhood. It was in the slave hospitals were American medical experimentation began.

Slave owners and physicians had a mutual level of understanding regarding slaves in the clinical process. A lot of physicians were slave owners themselves, which brought familiarity with handling sick slaves. It was the slave owner who gave or declined consent and responded in favor or disapproval to the physician. Slaves were not considered patients and deemed medically incompetent. Informed consent was ambiguous and often information was withheld if it complicated the medical process or left the slave paranoid.[36] However, there were rare occurrences of dual consent in the process of consent between the slave owner, physician, and slave.

Professor at Savanah Medical College, Dr. Juriah Harriss wanted to remove tumors from an enslaved woman's ears. Assuming that the tumors were no danger to the slave, the slave owner honored the slave woman's request.[37] In another example, Virginian surgeon Dr. Charles Bell Gibson was discerning his next move in a hernia operation of a slave man. The slave had an undescended testicle during the hernia surgery. Gibson decided not to remove the testicle because, "I had no right to castrate a man without his consent, or that of his master, prevailed against the temptation to lop off this misplaced testis."[38] Such form of graciousness should not be confused with the core of these decisions. The production of the slave was the most important result of these surgeries. Overall, slaves did not have ownership of their bodies, which made slaves vulnerable to surgical procedures and experimentations that caused them harm.

The third President of the United States of America, Thomas Jefferson, was a slave owner who fathered slaves. He was very interested in the field of medicine and often used his slaves as physical specimens for his clinical research. Specifically, Jefferson injected his slaves for vaccination experiments.[39] He was interested about the inoculation or variolation technique. In 1796, Dr. Edward Jenner created this technique injecting cowpox (disease of cattle) to establish immunity to smallpox. Hence, the inoculation process was injecting infected material from a sick person directly into a healthy person to induce immunity. Jenner discovered the localized and benign disease of cowpox when the disease was transmitted from the cow to human hands.[40] Jefferson used this technique on a slave who survived the inoculation process.

In 1832, the typhoid fever epidemic swept through Virginia. There was no cure for typhoid fever. Dr. Robert G. Jennings used the inoculation process on thirty slave and free blacks using the smallpox vaccine and withheld the vaccine from others. Jennings reported that his experiment worked.[41] Ironically, the smallpox vaccine is not efficacious against typhoid fever, but in Jenner's case miraculously worked. There has been no duplication and explanation on Jennings experiment, which remains a medical mystery. Through Jenner's technique, without any considered agency and consent, black slaves contributed to the acceptance of vaccination in American medicine.

Individuals classified as poor were used in experimentation. However, slaves' bodies were used to pursue clinical curiosity on how disease and illness works. Black bodies were used disproportionately more compared to other groups. Blacks had no legal protection from medical experimentation and no citizenship. Therefore, there were no consequences if a slave was abused or even killed for medical purposes. In the nineteenth and twentieth centuries, the black body was a figurine for medical research. For example, in 1836, half of the articles in the Southern Medical and Surgery Journal were on black bodies. For a second example, optometrist Dr. James Dugas used black slaves for 80% of the subjects of his pioneering eye technique. Lastly, slaves were used in genitourinary and bladder stone surgeries.[42]

The experimental usage of slave bodies was encouraged by the continued language by physicians that blacks did not feel pain or anxiety. Physicians like Dr. Charles White and Dr. James Johnson continued the discourse of black hardiness in the medical experimentation. Dr. White proclaimed, "[Blacks] bear surgical operations much better than white people and what would be the cause of insupportable pain for white men, a Negro would disregard… [I have] amputated the legs of many Negroes, who have held the upper part of the limb themselves."[43] Such an example of amputation was a slave who had a tenacious leg ulcer.

The slave's leg would not immediately respond to the medical staff's procedure, so the surgeon decided to cut the leg off. There were other possibilities, but the surgeon chose the most extreme option. The surgeon was reprimanded and was required to have to consult two professors in cases, "requiring an operation which may hazard the life of the patient or maim him."[44] It was rare, though, to see such a case of accountability for malpractice on a slave's body. It is possible that the medical staff was worried that the slave's owner would hold them liable destroying his property. Regardless, the perception of the surgeon's actions was due to the general notion of black durability in the medical community, which was promoted by Dr. Johnson.

Dr. Johnson was the editor of the influential *London Medical and Chirurgical Review*. Johnson stated, "When we come to reflect that all the women operated upon in Kentucky, except one, were Negresses and that these people will bear anything with nearly if not quite as much impunity as dogs and rabbits, our wonder is lessened."[45] Also, Dr. Thomas Hamilton, testing the idea of black heat tolerance, experimented on a slave named John Brown. Hamilton placed Brown into a makeshift open-pit oven trying to develop sunstroke medication. Brown stated that Hamilton, "Peeled off layers of his skin to determine how thick my black skin went."[46]

From 1846–1847, Dr. Walter F. Jones of Petersburg wanted to examine a cure for typhoid pneumonia. There was no exact number of individuals that were involved in the experiment, but the patients that were involved were black. One patient was a twenty-five-year-old slave. Jones explained,

> The patient was placed [naked] on the floor on his face, and about five gallons of water at a temperature so near the boiling point as barely to allow the immersion of the hand, was thrown immediately on the spinal column, which seemed to arouse his sensibilities somewhat, as shown by an effort to cry out; he was well rubbed and wrapped in blankets, and removed to bed. If necessary, the treatment was to be repeated in four hours.[47]

Jones asserted that many were cured from typhoid pneumonia by this technique that reestablished the capillary circulation of the patient. Overtime, Jones' procedure proved to be false.

One doctor that used medical experimentations that changed the physiological understanding of women and created the medical specialty gynecology was South Carolina born plantation physician J. Marion Sims. He believed in the idea of black durability. Literature like *The Biology of the Negro* and *SMJ*, influenced Sims perception of black women. The book states, "Women living under primitive conditions, as do most native Africans, go through pregnancy and delivery with comparative ease and little inconvenience."[48] In 1932, *SMJ* mentioned, "The colored woman because of her lessened sensibility to pain, is willing to endure a prolonged natural labor when a white woman would hours before be demanding relief."[49] Black women's "genital hardiness" was the justification of unanesthetized (no application of anesthesia) experimentations and influenced Sims's unanesthetized experimentations on slave women. For example, the introduction of the cesarean section procedure was very dangerous to the mother and infant. Enslaved women were used until the procedure was perfected and deemed harmless.[50]

Sims used eleven slaves to perform experimentations. His experimentations were not biased by sex. For example, Sims operated on a nineteen-year-old male slave, performing the unanesthetized removal of bone segments to prevent the spread of infection.[51] Sims infamous gynecological experiments took place in a Montgomery, Alabama with many subjects under the age of twenty. From 1845 to 1849, his experimentations were on slaves Anarcha, Betsey, Lucy, and others who suffered from vesico-vaginal fistula (VVF). VVF is an abnormal fistulous tract extending between the bladder and the vagina that allows the continuous involuntary discharge of urine into the vaginal vault.[52] VVF was a common condition for women in the nineteenth and twentieth century, with no bias towards a woman's socioeconomic status, that caused social isolation due to the atrocious odor it caused.

Sims invented the vaginal speculum, a device that opens the vaginal canal for medical examination.[53] His examination left slave women completely vulnerable with no sense of respect and privacy. Slave women were completely naked. Sims, prominent citizens, and local apprentices visually examined the women while several of his colleagues took turns inserting his speculum.[54] Sims declared, "I saw everything as no man had seen before."[55]

During his procedures, slave women were constrained to make incisions within the vagina. Sims never confirmed having performed a successful procedure for VVF, but most assumed he did. His colleague, assistant, critic Dr. Nathaniel Bozeman claimed he had to fix his VVF procedure in an occurrence when VVF was created by Sims removing bladder stones from a nine-year-old slave girl.[56] Sims was outraged and defended his successes correcting VVF. However, history of medicine tells us Sims was not the pioneer in VVF repair. In 1838, Virginian surgeon Peter Mettauer operated on twenty-five women in Prince Edward County, Virginia. Mettauer only cured one woman, and he cited the lack of intercourse prevention as the reason his women subjects did not heal.[57]

Sims and other physicians abused black slaves to explore bodily reactions to drugs and procedures, causing physical and psychological harm. The race-based idea of black hardiness falsely justified acts of maleficence because black individuals were considered different beings who really could handle the pain. Furthermore, the notion of black hardiness sustained the contradiction that black bodies were inferior and simultaneously physically superior. The trend of "hardy" black bodies being a tool for experimentation was continued in the United States military.

Military Experimentation

In World War II, the United States Office of Scientific Research and Development (OSRD) Army's Chemical Warfare Service and the Naval Research Laboratory conducted mustard gas experiments on 60,000 American Soldiers with at least nine race-based research projects based on race, pigment, and complexion.[58] Physicians wanted to determine African Americans, Asians (Japanese), and Hispanics' (Puerto Ricans') susceptibility to and injury from mustard gas, with whites being the control group. The involuntary experiments, in which it was considered one's patriotic honor to participate, were based on preparatory measures in case soldiers had to prepare for chemical warfare.

The mustard gas experiments had three goals: to train American soldiers if they were attacked by mustard gas, to determine the effectiveness mustard gas had against the enemy, and to define racial differences biologically. This was accomplished by the evaluation of specific clothing, gas masks, and skin applications (ointments). In what was called a "drop test" or "patch test" mustard agent was applied to soldiers' bare skin, which caused immediate and severe eye injuries, burns, oozing sores and blistering on the face, hands, underarms, buttocks, and genitals, which resulted in "lung damage, psychological disorders, cancer, asthma, emphysema, cancer, asthma, emphysema, and eye problems, and blindness."[59] Other known tests were "field tests" and "man-break tests." In the field tests, soldiers were sprayed with mustard gas wearing different forms of protective clothing and scientists who organized the man-break tests placed soldiers in mustard gas chambers to examine their stamina before incapacitation.[60] The mustard gas experiments were tools to confirm racial difference. Jim Crow law influenced the military's treatment of minorities and where experiments involving minorities took place.

African American, Japanese American, and Hispanic American units were segregated. At least, four research projects compared mustard gas exposure in African American soldiers and Japanese American soldiers to white soldiers.[61] African American and Hispanic men were used for defensive purposes. Black and Hispanic men's susceptibility to mustard gas (compared to white men) would determine their function on the front lines. The tests on Japanese Americans were for offensive purposes.

Such experiments were conducted at Cornell University Medical College, the University of Chicago Toxicity Laboratory, the Institute for Medical Research in Cincinnati, and the Rockefeller Institute for Medical Research.[62] Cornell University suggested racial differences in mustard gas exposure. Cornell stated, "All investigators agree that the skin of Negroes [sic] as a group is much less sensitive to mustard gas than the skin of whites. About 78 per cent of negroes [sic] are 'resistant' as compared with 20–40 per cent among the whites."[63] Cornell's rationale for its finding was the ingrained appropriations of blacks having thicker skin. Ultimately, the 1946 report by the OSRD and the National Defense Research Council concluded that the racial testing of African Americans was not conclusive. Medical scientists did not mention racial categories in their conclusions, but admitted their experiments as social constructs. The scientists concluded, "Race provided little, if any, meaningful health information."[64] The mustard gas experiments were recently resurfaced by National Public Radio (NPR) and Public Broadcasting Service (PBS) in 2015.

In 1956, the Central Intelligence Agency (CIA) and US Army personnel implemented "Operation Big City." Operation Big City was a secret biological warfare experiment executed in numerous East Coast cities.[65]

It was in the CIA's interest to confirm if different lung disease causing fungi affected blacks more than whites. The fungi were applied in
employment areas which where dominantly occupied by black employees. The purpose of the experiment was, "within this [supply] system,
there are employed large numbers of laborers, including many Negroes,
whose incapacitation would seriously affect the operation of the supply
system."[66] Other fungal experiments happened in the California Valley
and affected blacks and Asians, which also resulted in minorities more
susceptible to fungal infection than whites. The fungi experiments have
not been acknowledged by the US government. The US government
continued experimentation through plutonium experiments.

During World War II, Ebb Cade, a fifty-three-year-old African
American, worked as a cement mixer at the secret weapons production
plant in Oak Ridge, Tennessee. Cade got into an automobile accident
on his way to work, which resulted in a cut lip and nose and a fractured
right kneecap, forearm, left femur, and thigh bone.[67] He was kept at
the Manhattan Engineer District Hospital (Oak Ridge Army Hospital)
in Oak Ridge, Tennessee. Cade (known as patient HP-12) was injected
(without consent) with 4.7 out of 5 micrograms of plutonium by Los
Alamos chemist Wright Langham.[68] Cade's dosage is considered low,
but the lack of consent makes his case notorious. Plutonium is a highly
toxic element being purified to make atomic bombs.

Cade was thoroughly monitored with his dosage purposely imitating
the emission ratio in a lab worker. His blood, bone, urine, and stool
examined within hours of his plutonium injection. Cade's fifteen teeth
decayed and were pulled out for sampled plutonium. He was the first
out of eighteen subjects who were a part of a plutonium experiment in
the federally sponsored Manhattan Project, under contract to the US
Atomic Energy Commission (AEC).[69]

The Manhattan Project was the code name given to the program to
build an atomic bomb. The AEC succeeded the Manhattan Project. It
was involved in the development of atomic energy and created legislation for radiation research with human subjects. Blacks accounted for
60% of the human subjects in the Manhattan Project.[70] The purpose
of the plutonium experiments was to test the toxicity of this radioactive
chemical element. Other recorded plutonium subjects were,

> A 68-year-old man with advanced cancer of the mouth and lung became the second subject. Then a 55-year-old woman with breast cancer was injected ... and a young man with Hodgkin's disease on the same day, possibly at another Chicago area hospital. The older man with cancer received only 6.5 micrograms, but the breast cancer patient and the man with Hodgkin's disease received 95 micrograms.[71]

The excretion ratio turned out to be less than animals, which made the examination of stool from the plutonium subjects an inadequate means to determine a person's physiological reaction to plutonium. Due to the infamous nature of this experiment, the AEC neglected the word plutonium and used the code terms "product" or "49."[72] The plutonium projects were continued with Elmer Allen.

Elmer Allen was a thirty-six-year-old African American railroad porter for the Pullman Company. Allen hurt his knee from awkwardly falling off a train. His knee fracture would not heal. The Pullman Company would not accept liability for his injury, fired him, and did not give him any compensation. After dealing with his knee fracture and unemployment, Allen went to the University of California's clinic in San Francisco (UCSF).[73] Physicians concluded the reason his knee fracture would not heal was a result of chondrosarcoma (bone cancer).[74]

Allen needed his left knee amputated. After his amputation, Allen (known as patient CAL-3) was injected with plutonium. Allen was injected with more toxic plutonium called "plutonium-238" compared to the eighteen subjects injected with "plutinoim-239."[75] He was the only subject given a consent form, but full veracity and competency of the experiments was not disclosed. He was the last plutonium subject and outlived all the plutonium subjects who died to causes not related to the plutonium experiments. Allen died in 1991 due to pneumonia. Radiation trials were not the only experiments done on black bodies. Irradiation experiments were also popular in the mid-twentieth century.

University of Cincinnati's radiologist Eugene Saenger spearheaded the Total Body Irradiation (TBI) experiments. From 1960 to 1971, contracts between the University of Cincinnati and the Defense Atomic Support Agency did experiments: "People with 'radio-resistant' tumors were irradiated if there was thought to be a chance of benefit to them and to learn about how the treatment effected them, especially psychological and psychiatric effects."[76] The purpose was both palliative and informational for military treatment in defense situations.

The first patient was a sixty-seven-year-old black man with a cancer tumor on his left tonsil, which spread to his palate and throat. The sixty-seven-year-old did not survive. A total of 200 subjects participated in the TBI experiments with 75% or 150 being African American.[77] None of the subjects were aware of the risks like bone marrow suppression and nausea. Saenger never mentioned the side effects to the subjects and in any experiment documentation. Consent was verbal with no record of what the subjects were told.

African Americans were not the only racial groups that participated in race-based experiments, but they were the most used, sought after, and endured the worst experiments. Such factors harmed black soldiers who already sacrificed their well-being and livelihood to fight for a country that would not fight for them in return. The military's race-based experiments created maleficence to black soldiers' bodies which affected their autonomy. Many of the black soldiers' physiological capacities and quality of life diminished due to the physical strain of experimentation. Military race-based experimentation opened different avenues for institutions to conduct experiments. The next area of race-based experimentation happened in the prison system.

Prison Experimentation

Holmesburg Prison in Philadelphia, Pennsylvania conducted abusive experiments (tests) on its inmates, from the 1950s to the 1970s. The tests were led by dermatologist Dr. Albert M. Kligman. His research was on black and white men, but most of his research was done on black men. For example, the dioxin experiments had 49 black inmates compared to 9 white inmates.[78] Kligman did experiments for Johnson & Johnson, Merck, Helena Rubenstein, Dupont, and many others.[79] After World War II (WWII), the United States was the only country allowing experiments done on its prison population. Many cosmetic and pharmaceutical companies capitalized from Kligman's decades of research.

In the early 1960s, Al Zabala, a white twenty-seven-year-old Philadelphian, was serving a sentence for burglary. His penalty was enforced at Holmesburg Prison in Philadelphia, Pennsylvania. Prisoners, like Zabala, could not survive without money. Employment in prison did not provide a lot of options. Your choices were jobs in maintenance, custodial, kitchen, library staff (if the prison had one) and other menial jobs. The compensation was not adequate for daily survival, but becoming a test subject allowed opportunities for better compensation. At first, Zabala did not want to participate in the test, but it was hard for him to resist. Zabala said, "It was something to do, the best game in town. The money was good, and the money was easy."[80] The tests allowed Zabala to make quick and adequate money, an idea that attracted many prisoners.

The usual prison worker pay was 15 cents per day, but being a test subject was so much more financially beneficial. Zabala went through numerous of tests that comprised of him using foot powder, deodorant, creams, and shampoos. The compensation for foot powder and deodorant tests was $100 per month and hand cream tests were a $1 a day.[81] At that time, the prisoners felt the financial benefit outweighed the physical consequences. Zabala was a part of a test in which he believes he was injected with a substance ten times the potency of Lysergic Acid Diethylamide (LSD) and was monitored for seven days. Zabala described his experience,

> I wasn't right for a month after the test. I was real subdued and quiet. I had problems swallowing food and a constantly dry throat. They put me on a liquid diet until I could swallow whole food again. When we finally came back to the population, all the guys on the study had to wear badges that said we were no responsible for our actions and if we acted up to get U of P personnel to come and get us. We had to wear badges for a month and once a week talked to the psychs. They made us take paperwork and association tests to measure our psychological condition.[82]

Other prisoners who were subjects of the test experienced horrible hallucinations, trouble sustaining consciousness, self-violence, and violent temper tantrums.

Another experience recorded was that of black boxer Roy "Tiger" Williams. He served a 9–23 month sentence. Williams used an inmate named Sigmund Weitzman's shampoo. Weitzman was using "hair lotion" given to inmates who volunteered to test the product. Williams became bald stating, "The lotion removed my hair and anything else I had on my head."[83] Zabala's experience, though not ideal in any means, was better than the black inmates. Black inmates were treated with immense bias.

Black inmates did not get the desirable tests and received lower pay compared to the white inmates.[84] Kligman tested 153 different types of substances between 1962 and 1966 on 75% of Holmesburg Prison inmates.[85] Most of the experiments done on African Americans had to do with their skin. Similar to the mustard gas experiments, Klingman was influenced by Jim Crow law. He created protocols that ordered racially separated experiments. Kligman specifically designated certain experiments for black and white men. For example, a 1957 experiment was,

> Designed to promote the inoculation of human skin with … ectodermotropic viruses such as wart virus… herpes simplex and herpes zoster was reserved for healthy, colored, male volunteers between the ages of 20 and 45 years of age. Another is experimental inflammation and inflammatory dermatoses targeted 10 healthy white subjects who were paid to submerge one arm in a sodium lauryl sulfate solution one hour a day for 55 days in a row.[86]

Such skin experiments fortified the idea of the thickness of black skin. Other studies of black epidermis continued.

In a 1967 *Journal of Investigative Dermatology's* article, Klingman's sodium lauryl sulfate (SLS) and sodium tetrachloro-phenol (STP) experiments were documented. His findings suggest that SLS and STP were the best hardening agents for skin. Klingman concluded, "the solid hardening is attainable only if the skin passes through a very intense inflammatory phase with swelling, redness, scaling, and crusting."[87] These experiments were excruciatingly painful and permanently discolored and disfigured black inmates' skin. SLS and STP experiments concluded that "the Negro is more resistant to irritation."[88] In 1971, Klingman conducted a staph infection study with 150 inmates from twenty-five years old to forty years old. Most of the tests' subjects were African American. Only three inmates became ill, but the experiment cause lesions to form on inmates.

Holmesburg Prison's significant legal problem was the W-2429 experiment. A total of nine black subjects between twenty-three years old and thirty-one years old were involved in testing the safety and tolerance of Wallace Laboratories' W-2429 medication. One of the subjects, Jerome Roach, became ill four days after digesting temperature pills with a "sore throat, sore joints, fever, nausea, sores, and rashes."[89] Roach did not receive adequate treatment from the prison physician, which resulted in him being taken to Philadelphia General Hospital. Roach stayed at Philadelphia General Hospital for several weeks. He found out that his illness was a result of different pills given to him from those prescribed. When Roach returned to Holmesburg Prison, he was denied sufficient medical treatment and medication. As a result, Roach sued Klingman, but did not win the case because the court felt he was not "coerced" to be a part of the W-2429 experiment. The Holmesburg Prison was not the only criminal institution to conduct medical experiments. Sloan-Kettering Institute also conducted tests on prison inmates.

In 1952, Sloan-Kettering Institute's cancer tests were sponsored by the National Institutes of Health (NIH). Sloan's Dr. Chester M. Southam injected over 180 black Ohio State Prison's inmates with live human cancer cells.[90] Southam's objective was to see how a healthy human body would react to cancer cells. He was interested to see how cancer cells were neutralized and killed in healthy subjects. Southam did not disclose the full risk of the experiments to the black inmates.

From 1967 to 1969, Kilby, Draper, and McAlester prisons conducted blood-plasma trials in Alabama. The trials purpose was to test blood transfusions by using large quantities of plasma. Dr. Austin R. Stough managed the experiments. He was criticized because the experiments were disorganized with no informed consent or accurate records. Also, Stough's management also failed to keep the area of experiments clean. The disorganization and unsterile process of the blood-plasma trials led to inmates' sickness and death. Twenty-eight percent of subjects developed hepatitis.[91] Many subjects (black and white) died because of the unsterile trial areas and blood transfusions of the wrong blood type.

Another incident of prison experiments was at Tulane University. In the 1950s, Tulane University conducted psycho surgery experiments (funded by the CIA) on black inmates with no informed consent. Tulane psychiatrist Robert Heath purposely selected black subjects to participate in experiments. Heath's experiments involved inserting electrodes into subjects' brains to stimulate the part of the brain that transmits pleasure.[92] Also, Heath and Harry Bailey (Heath's assistant) participated in trials using LSD and bulbocapnine at Louisiana State Penitentiary. The LSD and bulbocapnine affected an individual's faculties and cognition, which was used to control violent prisoners. The experiments were conducted exclusively on black inmates with no informed consent. The CIA wanted to collect data on the two substances if induced, resulted in, "loss of speech, loss of sensitivity to pain, loss of memory, loss of will power and an increase in toxicity in persons with a weak type of central nervous system."[93] The LSD experiment was an example of how race-based experimentation in the prison system aided in understanding how bodies react to certain diseases and procedures.

The use of black prisoners was very popular in race-based experimentation in prisons. Many of the prisoners died before being released or had a poor quality of life that affected their daily autonomy. Such prison and military experiments happened after a global consensus to stop unethical treatment on human subjects.

International Codes and Ethical Standards

The Nuremberg Code and the Declaration of Helsinki are useful tools for examining how research on human beings should be conducted. In 1947, The Nuremberg Code (also known as the Doctors' Trial) was a series of ten principles developed by American judges who responded to Nazi doctors who conducted human experiments on concentration camp inmates.[94] It is the foundational blueprint that set the precedent for principles on human subjects involved in experiments and medical research.

In 1964, the Declaration of Helsinki was adopted by the World Medical Association. It was constructed to, "meet the threat that inappropriate research posed both to the integrity and the reputation of the research enterprise."[95] It added three significant factors to the Nuremberg Code. The distinction between clinical therapeutic research and nontherapeutic biomedical research, an advocacy mechanism to enforce that the principles are followed, and the proxy consent by family members when the subject cannot consent.[96] It is imperative that the highest level of efficacy in research be used for the improvement of the human condition.

The experiments mentioned previously (except for slave experiments) were conducted after these ethical laws were in place.[97] The absence of compliance and penalties for experiments specifically on African Americans showed how the legacy of race-based experimentation influenced ongoing medical practices. American medicine created laws they did not follow and mocked the value of clinical ethics. Allowing such treatment of African Americans was a violation of internationally agreed upon commitments.

Research ethics emphasize respecting the autonomy of participants. It is the commitment to "building up or maintaining others' capacities for autonomous choice while helping to allay fears and other conditions that destroy or disrupt autonomous actions."[98] The realities of military and prison experiments on black bodies did the complete opposite. Research was performed without informed voluntary consent of participants. To be balanced, informed consent was not even thought of until the late 1950s and put into examination of clinical trials until the early 1970s.[99] However, due to sustained racist perceptions, black bodies were not granted equal consideration.

Informed consent allows patients or participants to be aware of the "nature and results (the potential risks and benefits) of each course of actions open to them before they make their decision."[100] Military and prison experiments did not disclose any potential risks and benefits, thus violating informed consent, a key procedure in the clinical process. Specifically, prison experiments were coercive, using monetary means to attract participants. To be clear, monetary incentive can be a useful means to compensate participants for their involvement in trials. The ethical issue with the mentioned prison experiments was that corporate gain was the reason for participants' involvement in trials.

Adequate compensation was a challenge for prisoners. The prison and clinical trial directors knew about the prisoners' financial struggles and used monetary resources to get participants. Informed consent minimizes the chance that people will be deceived, exploited, tricked, misled, duped, manipulated, or pressured so that their autonomy is violated.[101] Informed consent was not used because the prisoners' autonomy and decision making was violated through monetary means. Another issue was the lack of consideration given to measuring the risks and gains of trials.

In clinical trials, the participants' gains anticipated from the experiment must be commensurate with the risks. The results of loss, injury, and deformation of prisoner participants completely outweighed the gains of the prison trials. Similar results were found with the military trials. The prisoner and military experiments were nontherapeutic biomedical research which solely had scientific value for the researchers. Yet, the ethical issues with the military and prison experiments were that the special interest of a few took precedence over the well-being of the participants.

Military and prison experimentation did not follow the ethical commitments required in clinical trials. The codes and declarations of conduct in research without proper enforcement do a disservice to such policies themselves. The autonomy of participants are manipulated and unacknowledged, which hinders the outcome of non-maleficence, beneficence, and justice being practiced. Other racial groups were involved in military and prison experiments, but blacks endured the worst procedures. As a result, there are core consequences that developed in the black community.

Black Community's Response to Race-Based Experimentation

For centuries, race-based experimentations used the black body to explore biological and physiological understanding for medical progression. This unique medical history of minorities (especially African

Americans) created an uncomfortable relationship in medicine. It is logical to perceive that such histories of medical experiments on black individuals fractured the psyche of the black community's thoughts regarding and involvement in American medicine. African Americans reacted to these medical experiments by developing a language of distrust that has heavily impacted black oral tradition regarding medicine.

Black Oral Tradition

Oral tradition is a significant part in black culture. Tradition, ideas, and experiences are verbally passed down from generation to generation. Oral tradition is understood to be, "the transmission of cultural items from one member to another, or others. Those items are heard, *stored in memory*, and when appropriate, recalled at the moment of subsequent transmission" (emphasis added).[102] The realities of medical experimentation among African Americans became stories within oral tradition that are heard, stored, and recalled. When blacks individually and collectively interact with the clinical or medical process, the memories of mistreatment of friends, living family members, and predecessors are relived and processed. The black individual may not have experienced or lived medical experimentation, but still feel a sense of association because of their unique racial history in American society. The notion is not individual but collective. The thought was, "If it happened to him or her, it can happen to me."

Furthermore, oral tradition is a preservation mechanism.[103] Stories and experiences are preserved along with feelings and emotions. It is through such language that blacks developed their own view of reality and society. The oral tradition of African Americans is a product of their environment in medicine. It is a reminder of how medicine and society express and reflects itself toward African Americans. Such inhumane and racist medical treatment influenced blacks' distrust toward American medicine. Blacks' distrust of American medicine had its origins in slavery.

Black slaves' oral traditions reported the abuses of the black body on plantations. Slaves did not want to take what they called "white man's medicine" or "white medicine," because of anxiety and fear. Slaves acted like they were not sick, so they would not have to see white doctors and take white medicine. Slaveholders noticed the apprehension of blacks. A Mississippi planter said, "The Negroes unfortunately for themselves and equally so for us had no confidence in our treatment- they said it was certain death to take our medicine and we were compelled to stand by and see them die."[104] Slaves distrust heightened when they were forced to take white medicine or get punished.

It was always an issue for the slave to follow the white doctor's orders to take white medicine and stay in bed. Blacks did not want to go to slave hospitals or infirmaries, and often were forced to go as a last resort. A Richmond, Virginia newspaper commented,

> Among them there prevails superstition that when they enter the [medical college] infirmary they never come out alive; (although servants are no where better treated and taken care of than in that establishment;) therefore they will not complain, but will often conceal their real condition until too late to do good.[105]

This extremely contradictory statement by the Richmond newspaper suggests the historical disconnect between whites' understandings and slave's perception of care. If medical care was adequate, slaves would not be so reluctant to be treated at slave hospitals, infirmaries, and other medical establishments. The inhumane treatment and abuses experienced by slaves made it completely logical for them to avoid white medicine and clinics at all costs. The slaves' oral tradition of their experience and perception of American medicine influenced their participation in such a system. Through oral tradition, such experiences permeate blacks' memories. The historical strain American medicine has on blacks affects the group's language and understanding of care. Ultimately, American medicine's racist history resulted in blacks' poor health literacy.

Health literacy is not exclusive to reading and writing, but "the wide range of skills and competencies that people develop to seek out, comprehend, evaluate, and use health information and concepts to make informed choices, reduce health risks, and increase quality of life."[106] Health literacy at its core stresses veracity and probity, which blacks did not experience. However, these two qualities can change because health literacy is a continuing process. In the black community, oral tradition shapes one's health literacy. It informs the process and interaction of African Americans with American medicine and care.

As Dr. Christina Zarcadoolas suggests, "Health literacy evolves over one's lifetime and like most other complex human competencies, is affected by health status as well as demographic, sociopolitical, psychosocial, and cultural factors."[107] The 246 years of chattel slavery contained numerous lifetimes and generations of black slaves who did not have adequate health literacy or healthcare. Neither could be offered in those time periods because of a society and system that valued them as less than human. Such realities were passed down in black oral tradition. As a result, blacks had improper or no use of medication, no use of health services, poor self-management of chronic conditions, inadequate response in emergency situations, poor health outcomes, lack of self-efficacy and self-esteem, and social inequity.[108] In order to survive, blacks had to create their own system of treatments and medications to survive in a racist society.

Black Homeopathic Medicine

Black homeopathy (also known as homeopathic medicine) is a medical system that offers a variety of approaches to medicine (i.e. herbal, botanical, traditional, psychological, and spiritual).[109] Homeopathic medicine has been understood as a German development credited to German physician Samuel Hahnemann in the eighteenth century. However, homeopathy's origin dates to ancient African tribes who incorporated nature's surroundings as their physical and spiritual source of healing. Sacred power, spiritual healing and nature were used as collective processes of healing.

American homeopathy began with Native Americans and expanded with black slaves. Blacks and Native Americans were enslaved together and meshed their histories of homeopathy together.[110] Black homeopathy continued in the early to mid-seventeenth century by black slaves and Native Americans as a necessary method to survive the daily physical burden of slave work. Through the resource of oral tradition, blacks' home remedies, treatments, and plant and herb knowledge were passed generations as a response of self-preservation.

Plants like sesame, yams, okra, and black-eyed peas originated in Africa and were grown on American plantations. Slaves used licorice plants for coughs and fevers, okra leaves as poultices (soft moist mass) applied to the body to relieve soreness and inflammation, Jamaican senna as a laxative, "Surinam poison" for chronic sores, kola seeds for belly pains, mackaroot tea to cure worms, pepper/dogwood tea for fevers, snakeroot for stomach aches, and collard leaf as a cure for head-aches.[111] Blacks protected these medical traditions by secretly sharing with caution. White doctors only paid attention to black homeopa-thy when a slave made a great medical discovery. For example, a slave named Caesar received a 300 pound pension for treating poisoning and snake bites.[112]

Whites felt threatened by black homeopathy and viewed it as "native," "negro superstition," "voodoo," or "hoodoo."[113] There was a legitimate fear that black homeopathy and its spiritual elements would spread and challenge Christianity. As a response, in 1748, Virginia passed laws to prohibit blacks from practicing homeopathy. In 1749, South Carolina's general assembly passed a law prohibiting slaves from being employed by physicians and distributing treatment.[114] Regardless of these laws, whites used black homeopathy for treatment because they felt it was more efficacious compared to what white doctors had to offer. Slaveholders personally preferred black practitioners over whites. Slaves who had no human and citizen rights uniquely garnered medi-cal status by traditional knowledge of black homeopathy. Blacks became herbalists, practitioners, and doctors of botany (the science of plants) or "Negro Medicine." Black homeopathy revolutionized American phar-macopoeia (the making of drugs).

Blacks used botanicals for many purposes. Women used honeysuckle and rose petals as perfume, men used barks for belt, and children used twigs and whistle for games. Black herbalists believed blood quality was the key factor for diagnosis and an indicator of health status. Black herbalists used many remedies to purge out sickness in the blood. The most popular used was the sassafras root made into a tea. It was believed the tea, "searches de blood and finds out what's wrong and goes to work on it."[115] Such ingenuity and sophistication of African Americans' understandings of herbs, plants, and other resources challenged the status quo of black intellectual inferiority.

Blacks' dualistic reaction to atrocious clinical care and experiments sustained the oral tradition of fear and health illiteracy, but resulted in black homeopathy. Black homeopathy was the slaves reaction; a good consequence of unethical medical behavior. It made a racist medical system aware that African Americans and other minorities are valuable and can contribute to the progression of medicine. Black homeopathy became the medium of clinical justice, the means to participate and be heard in the clinical process. The misappropriations of black body and race-based experiments have left deep wounds in minority communities, but black homeopathy was a means of medical sanity.

Race-based medicine was the catalyst for treating the African Americans body as a different entity with unique functions. Such ideas promoted experimentations that critically fractured blacks' relationship with clinical care and physicians. However, black homeopathy began the process of African Americans' reconciliation and contribution to medicine. In Chapter 3, I will examine race-based medicine in its pharmaceutical form in a drug called BiDil, along with its history, development, approval, and the financial, scientific, genetic and racial tensions it produces. This chapter will further suggest solutions to race-based medicine through physicians perfecting their cultural competency, empathic communication, and awareness with a focus on diet and nutrition.

Notes

1. Hoberman, *Darwin's Athletes*, 150.
2. Holloway, Karla F. C. *Private Bodies, Public Texts: Race, Gender, and a Cultural Bioethics*. Durham, NC: Duke University Press, 2011, 9.
3. Ibid., 18.
4. Beauchamp, Tom, and James Childress. *Principles of Biomedical Ethics*, 6th ed. Oxford: Oxford University Press, 2008, 99.
5. Holloway, *Private Bodies, Public Texts*, 20.
6. Beauchamp and Childress, *Principles of Biomedical Ethics*, 103.

7. Such examples happened to sports legends Jesse Owens and Jackie Robinson. Owens and Robinson are among the first black professional athletes to be typecasted, scrutinized, and medically examined due to their athletic abilities. The "extra tendon" in black athletes' legs or sensitive heel that makes them jump higher or run faster than normal, are physiological misconceptions that still exist in our society. Owens and Robinson are examples of how American Society viewed African Americans as "the other" type of personhood.

8. Hoberman, *Darwin's Athletes*, 147.

9. Hoberman, *Darwin's Athletes*, 213.

10. Ibid., 185.

11. Nolen, Claude H. *The Negro's Image in the South: The Anatomy of White Supremacy*. Lexington: University of Kentucky Press, 1967, 3.

12. Hoberman, *Darwin's Athletes*, 188.

13. Hoberman, *Darwin's Athletes*, 176.

14. Ibid., 153.

15. Ibid., 158.

16. Ibid., 196.

17. Ibid., 200.

18. Hoberman, *Darwin's Athletes*, 194.

19. Ibid., 149.

20. Ibid., 148.

21. Hoberman, *Darwin's Athletes*, 150.

22. Ibid., 152–153.

23. Ibid., 174.

24. Nolen, *The Negro's Image in the South*, 5.

25. Hoberman, *Darwin's Athletes*, 176.

26. Ibid., 177.

27. Ibid., 183.

28. Covey, *African American Slave Medicine*, 44–45.

29. Dr. Davis' book explores resistance to scientific hegemony in nineteenth-century literature. She explains medical and scientific constructions of embodied identity were assigned to African Americans. Dr. Davis' work contributes to the conversation of how American medicine and medical literature sustains oppressive perceptions of black bodies.

30. Davis, Cynthia J. *Bodily and Narrative Forms: The Influence of Medicine on American Literature, 1845–1915*. Stanford, CA: Stanford University Press, 2000, 14.

31. Jackson, Ronald L. *Scripting the Black Masculine Body Identity, Discourse, and Racial Politics in Popular Media.* Albany: State University of New York Press, 2006, 18.
32. Holloway, *Private Bodies, Public Texts,* 114.
33. Washington, Harriet A. *Medical Apartheid: The Dark History of Medical Experimentation on Black Americans from Colonial Times to the Present.* New York: Doubleday, 2006, 55.
34. The most notorious examples of clinical or medical experimentation and treatment of African Americans were the Tuskegee Study of Untreated Syphilis in the Negro Male (also known as the Tuskegee Experiment) and Henrietta Lacks' cervical cancer tumor cells called "HeLa cells" being used for research and monetary gains. In both cases, black subjects were not given informed consent (an individual's autonomous authorization of a medical intervention or of participation of research) and were taken advantage of due to their socioeconomic status. The Tuskegee Experiment and Henrietta Lacks cases are examples of many medical abuses on the black body and are not the only cases of unethical treatment of minorities.
35. Washington, *Medical Apartheid,* 57.
36. Fett, *Working Cures,* 145.
37. Fett, *Working Cures,* 146.
38. Ibid.
39. Washington, *Medical Apartheid,* 59.
40. Savitt, Todd Lee. *Medicine and Slavery: The Diseases and Health Care of Blacks in Antebellum Virginia.* Urbana: University of Illinois Press, 1978, 294.
41. Washington, *Medical Apartheid,* 60.
42. Washington, *Medical Apartheid,* 57.
43. Ibid., 58.
44. Savitt, *Medicine and Slavery,* 288.
45. Washington, *Medical Apartheid,* 58.
46. Fett, *Working Cures,* 152.
47. Savitt, *Medicine and Slavery,* 299.
48. Hoberman, *Darwin's athletes,* 178.
49. Ibid.
50. Fett, *Working Cures,* 151.
51. Washington, *Medical Apartheid,* 63.
52. Savitt, *Medicine and Slavery,* 297.

53. Washington, *Medical Apartheid*, 64.
54. Ibid.
55. Ibid.
56. Ibid., 67.
57. Savitt, *Medicine and Slavery*, 298.
58. Smith, "Mustard Gas and American Race-Based," 517–518.
59. Smith, "Mustard Gas and American Race-Based," 518.
60. Ibid.
61. Ibid., 518–519.
62. Ibid., 519.
63. Ibid.
64. Smith, "Mustard Gas and American Race-Based," 520.
65. Washington, *Medical Apartheid*, 382–383.
66. Ibid., 383.
67. Welsome, Eileen. *The Plutonium Files: America's Secret Medical Experiments in the Cold War*. New York, NY: Dial Press, 1999, 83.
68. Moreno, Jonathan D. *Undue Risk: Secret State Experiments on Humans*. New York: W.H. Freeman, 2000, 124–125.
69. Welsome, *The Plutonium Files*, 84.
70. Washington, *Medical Apartheid*, 219.
71. Moreno, *Undue Risk*, 126.
72. Washington, *Medical Apartheid*, 219.
73. Moreno, *Undue Risk*, 124–134.
74. Washington, *Medical Apartheid*, 221.
75. Ibid.
76. Moreno, *Undue Risk*, 212.
77. Washington, *Medical Apartheid*, 233.
78. Hornblum, Allen M. *Acres of Skin: Human Experiments at Holmesburg Prison: A True Story of Abuse and Exploitation in the Name of Medical Science*. New York: Routledge, 1998, 171.
79. Washington, *Medical Apartheid*, 249.
80. Hornblum, *Acres of Skin*, 5–6.
81. Ibid., 6.
82. Ibid., 7.
83. Hornblum, *Acres of Skin*, 13.
84. Ibid., 17.
85. Washington, *Medical Apartheid*, 249.
86. Hornblum, *Acres of Skin*, 17.

87. Hornblum, *Acres of Skin*, 144.

88. Ibid., 145.

89. Ibid., 201.

90. Washington, *Medical Apartheid*, 252.

91. Ibid., 253.

92. Washington, *Medical Apartheid*, 254.

93. Ibid.

94. Brody, Baruch A. *The Ethics of Biomedical Research: An International Perspective*. New York: Oxford University Press, 1998, 33.

95. Ibid., 34.

96. Ibid.

97. Slave experiments happened centuries before international codes were created. Therefore, it is not feasible to include slave experiments in this section.

98. Beauchamp and Childress, *Principles of Biomedical Ethics*, 103.

99. Ibid., 117.

100. Steinbock, Bonnie. *The Oxford Handbook of Bioethics*. Oxford University Press on Demand, 2007, 218.

101. Ibid., 217.

102. Mugalu, Joachim. *Philosophy, Oral Tradition and Africanistics: A Survey of the Aesthetic and Cultural Aspects of Myth, with a Case-Study of the "Story of Kintu" from Buganda (Uganda), as a Contribution to the Philosophical Investigations in Oral Traditions*. Frankfurt am Main: Peter Lang, 1995, 54.

103. Ibid., 56.

104. Fett, *Working Cures*, 147–148.

105. Savitt, *Medicine and Slavery*, 283.

106. Zarcadoolas, Christina, Andrew F. Pleasant, and David S. Greer. *Advancing Health Literacy: A Framework for Understanding and Action*. San Francisco, CA: Jossey-Bass, 2006, 5–6.

107. Ibid., 55.

108. Zarcadoolas, et al., *Advancing Health Literacy*, 1–2.

109. Covey, *African American Slave Medicine*, 42.

110. Fett, *Working Cures*, 64.

111. Fett, *Working Cures*, 63–71.

112. Covey, *African American Slave Medicine*, 44.

113. Ibid.

114. Ibid., 43.

115. Fett, *Working Cures*, 75.

4

Research, Race and Profit

Health disparity based on racial categories has been a popular topic for quite some time. Health challenges among American minority populations are no secret. Individuals within Black, Hispanic, and Asian communities are the most disadvantaged regarding well-being. The use of Pharmacology (the branch of medicine focusing on the knowledge and study of drugs) is a tool to alleviate health issues in minority communities. Specifically, heart failure is a major American public health issue. Compared to other races, African Americans suffer disproportionately higher rates of heart failure. Consequently, BiDil was designed to specifically treat African Americans, which made BiDil the first drug categorized as race-based medicine. This chapter will examine significant heart studies before BiDil, BiDil's path to approval and the racial aftershock felt in the areas of economics, medicalization, and genetics with physician-patient critiques and nutritional solutions.

© The Author(s) 2019
K. A. Johnson, *Medical Stigmata*,
https://doi.org/10.1007/978-981-13-2992-0_4

Before BiDil

Up until the mid-twentieth century, there were studies regarding the effects of cardiovascular disease, but not its causes. The three types of heart disease, categorized in 1928, were rheumatic, syphilitic, and arteriosclerotic.[1] In 1948, the United States Public Health Service (USPHS) (formally known as the National Heart Institute (NHI) and currently called the National Heart, Lung, and Blood Institute (NHLBI)) began an important study within the arena of cardiology. The USPHS partnered with the Massachusetts Department of Health and Harvard's Department of Preventative Medicine to create the Framingham Heart Study (FHS).[2] Cardiovascular studies before FHS identified factors of cardiovascular disease after the patient already had it. The purpose of the FHS study was, "To study the expression of coronary artery disease in a normal or unselected population and determine the factors *predisposing* to the development of the disease through laboratory experimentation and long-term follow up of such a group" (emphasis added).[3]

FHS was based out of Framingham, Massachusetts (population of 28,000 in 1949) with 5209 patients all white men and women between the ages of 30–62 with children added later in 1971.[4] It is important to note none of these patients had serious symptoms of cardiovascular disease and did not have prior cardiovascular episodes (i.e. heart attack or stroke). The patients' follow up spanned a five to ten year period. FHS' goal was to find connections between the patients' lifestyles, test results, and heart disease, which set the precedent for how future studies would eventually conduct measures for cardiovascular disease factors.

Initially, doctors in the mid-twentieth century suggested stress was a factor that can contribute to illness. The medical mindset of that time understood the heart as an important organ reflecting the cause and management of stress. The daily demands in modernity caused stress on the heart and the tool of medicine can alleviate cardiac stressors. FHS supporter Dr. Paul Dudley White, the Father of American Cardiology, asserted, "stress and strain" in modern times should not be overlooked, but should be an essential piece in learning more about cardiovascular disease.[5] White's exploration of cardiovascular disease was rooted in his understanding of race.

Cardiovascular disease was not an African American issue, but a white issue. In 1921, twenty seven years before FHS, Dr. Haven Emerson reported to the Massachusetts Medical Society, "The white race is more susceptible to heart disease than the colored race."[6] Furthermore, in 1930, University of Pennsylvania's Dr. C. C. Wolferth asserted to the *New York Times*, "Degenerative diseases of the heart and blood vessels comprise what is probably the most important problem facing the *white race*" (emphasis added).[7] Even Dr. Paul Dudley White claimed that a "full-blooded Negro"[8] did not get cardiovascular disease. However, there were rare arguments by individuals like Drs. Edward Schwab and Victor Schulze who suggested African Americans had more heart disease and higher mortality rates than whites.[9] Cardiology and modernity were linked by racial discourse which brought a narrative that stress was associated with "whiteness."

Dr. Stewart R. Roberts who was the Professor of Clinical Medicine at Emory University (1915–1941), President of the Southern Medical Society (1924–1925), and President of the American Heart Association (AHA) (1933–1934) compared whites as stressed and African Americans as joyous and carefree. Roberts said,

> The white man, particularly those living lives of stress in urban conditions of competition, work and strain, makes his little plains and layups cares and riches and takes much thought of the morrow; the negro knows his weekly wage is his fortune, takes each day as it is, takes little or no thought of the morrow, plays, and lives in a state of play, hurries none and worries little. What must it be to live unhurried, unworried, superstitious but not ambitious, full of childlike faith, satisfied, helpless, plodding, plain, patient, yet living a life of joy and interest?[10]

The founding fathers of cardiology profoundly influenced the medical narrative of cardiovascular disease by their racial discourse. Cardiology titans like Emerson, Wolferth, White, and Roberts created a medical narrative that constructed white individuals as victims of stress by a societal burden of responsibility, while establishing African Americans as the bystanders in societal progress.

Roberts diagnosed this societal burden as "neurasthenia." Neurasthenia is a late nineteenth century term that described physical and mental fatigue, dizziness, headaches, bodily pains, concentration difficulties, sleep disturbance, and memory loss.[11] Neurasthenia was an epidemiological persuasion of "the white man's burden," a disorder that was the result of the heavy weight of responsibility whites had for the sake of American progress.

A key evaluation about the FHS, cardiovascular disease and modernity was solely based on the representation of "white" individuals as human subjects. FHS' "diversity" was described by the European location of the patients (i.e. England, Italy, Poland, Greece, Ireland, and French Canada). The exclusion of African Americans in clinical research was not out of the ordinary. As a matter of medical and historical fact, African Americans clinical exclusion was normal. As discussed in Chapter 1, eugenic influences on race ideology and perception influenced the medical world's view of African Americans' personhood, to which cardiology was not an exception. Eugenic logic dismissed individuals that were viewed as "less than human" and lacked human agency in clinical research and focus on individuals who were viewed as "genetically fit" to be the legitimate representation of American society. African American mortality was not viewed as important for the progression of modernity, an idea that was emphasized in early cardiology practice.

FHS' influence is unprecedented. FHS spearheaded the emphasis of the 1960s risk factor approach in the medical community. The term "risk factor" was first used in a FHS investigators' report in 1961 and the core of new heart related research in the late twentieth and twenty first century was based from FHS.[12] FHS findings suggested the factors of cardiovascular disease were caused by physiologic function (body function), poor diet, family history, individual behavior, high blood pressure, diabetes mellitus (different types of diabetes), genetics, and hyperlipidemia (abnormally high concentration of fats or lipids in the blood).[13] These findings show that there are numerous factors that may cause cardiovascular disease. FHS' introduction of risk factors did not only open the medicine world's eyes to aid in the prevention of cardiovascular disease, but led to inquiries about the unknown risk factors of other diseases.

In the 1970s, hydralazine and isosorbide dinitrate (H/I) were discovered as key ingredients in drugs used to fight against heart failure and cardiovascular disease. In the 1970s, two Veterans Administration Cooperative Studies known as Vasodilator Heart Failure Trial (V-HeFT) I and II. V-HeFT I were developed and implemented from 1980–1985. The patient population of V-HeFT I came from many racial backgrounds comprised of people who already took digoxin and a diuretic. The participants were broken into three groups by random selection. Group one received a placebo, group two received prazosin, and group three received the H/I combination. The findings suggested the placebo and prazosin were not effective. However, the investigators of V-HeFT I concluded that the H/I combination was an "effective new treatment for heart failure regardless of race."[14] The V-HeFT I trial laid the foundation for the V-HeFT II trial.

The V-HeFT II trial (1986–1991) compared the H/I combination to an angiotensin-converting enzyme (ACE) inhibitor called enalapril. ACE inhibitors widen or dilate blood vessels to improve the amount of blood flow the heart pumps, which helps to decrease the amount of work a heart must do. Also, ACE inhibitors help in lowering blood pressure. The findings suggest the enalapril group had a positive mortality rate, but the H/I combination group yielded numerous results because the H/I combination's efficacy and side effects varied. The findings were confirmed in a report asserting, "20 per cent to 30 per cent of congestive heart failure patients do not respond favorably to standard therapies of diuretics, digitals or ACE inhibitors… particularly ACE inhibitors."[15] Medical discourse on risk factors continued to permeate through the twentieth century through the Jackson Heart Study (JHS) in 1987.

The JHS emerged out of concern by the founder of the Association of Black Cardiologists (ABC) Dr. Richard Allen Williams, for long-term observation of cardiovascular risk factors. Williams challenged the relevance of FHS in the African American community and wanted an African American version of FHS. JHS materialized from the multi-community study named Atherosclerosis in Communities (ARIC), in Jackson Mississippi. The ARIC study had 5302 "self-identified" African American patients between the ages of 35–84 years old.[16] The JHS patients' information was embedded in a genetic collection for future study. JHS' patients came from a participant lottery, the ARIC program and volunteers from the Jackson, Mississippi area.

JHS's goal was to illustrate similarities of blacks and whites and discredit the naïve notion that only blacks get hypertension and are immune to cardiovascular disease. JHS, also known as the "Black Framingham," did not want to create a medical narrative that African Americans were biologically different from other racial groups, but wanted to break the racial glass ceiling in clinical research asserting African Americans are viable human beings capable of representing humanity. JHS set the precedence for minority inclusion for serious consideration in quantitative analysis in clinical research, which influenced the passing of the National Institutes of Health (NIH) Revitalization Act of 1993 which required, "federally funded clinical trials include women and ethnic minorities as subjects and disaggregate statistics by gender and ethnicity."[17] Before the development of JHS, the city of Jackson's ARIC program represented the largest historical effort to recruit African Americans in clinical research.[18] JHS results show important factors like socioeconomic status and psychosocial elements profoundly impact African Americans' heart health. JHS's findings urged a medical solidarity for cardiovascular disease in the African American community. The development of a race-based drug was constructed to be the solution for African Americans with heart failure.

BiDil's Beginnings

In 1989, V-HeFT's lead cardiologist and University of Minnesota professor, John Cohn received a non-racial patent of the H/I combination improving heart treatments. In 1992, BiDil ("Bi" meaning two and "Dil" meaning dilators), the H/I combination into one pill, was filed as a new drug. In 1995, Medco (pharmacy benefit manager "PBM" who process and pay drug claims) received patent rights from Cohn and trademarked BiDil. In 1996, Medco attempted to get the Food & Drug Administration's (FDA) approval for BiDil which was denied, in a nine to three decision, due to unclear data in V-HeFT trial. The V-HeFT trials' data did not meet regulatory statistical standards to establish efficacy for the new drug. The FDA asserted, "V-HeFT I and II trials had to be stopped prematurely due to funding problems. They therefore did not have sufficient power for their planned [statistical] analyses."[19] Medco gave up the patent process and returned the intellectual property rights of BiDil to Cohn.

After BiDil's first rejection by the FDA, Cohn analyzed data by race. Cohn used old data from the V-HeFT I and II trials which compared 395 African Americans with 1024 whites. The only remote racial difference shown was in the V-Heft I trial with only 49African Americans taking the H/I combination. According to Cohn, "The H/I combination appears to be particularly effective in prolonging survival in black patients and is as effective as enalapril in this subgroup. By contrast, enalapril shows its more favorable effect on survival, particularly in the white popula-tion."[20] Cohn's findings was published in an article "Racial Differences in Response to Therapy for Heart Failure: Analysis of the Vasodilator-Heart Failure Trials,"[21] asserting BiDil functions better in African Americans compared to whites. The article was a key factor in the FDA's approval.

The article asserted racial groups might have different reactions to drugs. Cohn and Carson asserted a specific drug had the probabil-ity to react in different ways among racial groups. The article also laid the foundation for using BiDil as a drug treatment for heart failure in African Americans. The momentum of the article caused Cohn to rel-icense BiDil and give the production rights to NitroMed. NitroMed licensed the same H/I combination for a non-race-specific patent from 1987 to 2007 and an African American patent from 2000 to 2020. NitroMed continued to gain momentum for BiDil and raised over $30 million to start their African-American Heart Failure Trial (A-HeFT).[22]

FDA's Approval

In the A-HeFT trial (2004), follow-up was planned for 18 months 1050 "self-identified African-Americans" were subjects. NitroMed's Data Safety Monitoring Board stopped the A-HeFT trial because of the discovery that "BiDil reduced mortality rates by some 43%,"[23] which NitroMed felt was a sufficient percentage. In June 2005, the FDA approved BiDil as a drug to treat African Americans with heart failure. BiDil made history as the first race-based drug. The FDA had four justifications for approving BiDil. The FDA asserted,

> (1) Data from 3 clinical trials showed dramatic effectiveness of hydralazine hydrochloride and isosorbide dinitrate in black patients and supported a differential effect in black and white patients. (2) Not understanding the reasons for the difference in treatment effect by race did not justify withholding the treatment from those who could benefit from it. (3) Regulatory and other concerns associated with drug approval for narrow patient populations did not justify withholding BiDil from those who could benefit from it. (4) Race and other demographic characteristics have long been important to consider in analysis of trials and as a matter of equity and justice.[24]

From the FDA's perspective, these reasons justified the approval of BiDil as an important element in the alleviation of heart failure in the African American population. However, the FDA did not ignore the inconsistencies of NitroMed's clinical trials.

FDA's Justifications

The FDA's first justification for approving BiDil created controversy because its clinical trials had no other racial populations to compare results to, which left BiDil's African American efficacy uncertain. The FDA asserted, "Data from 3 clinical trials showed dramatic effectiveness of hydralazine hydrochloride and isosorbide dinitrate in black patients and supported a differential effect in black and white patients."[25] For decades, H/I has helped black and white patients with heart failure and cardiovascular disease. FDA's affirmation that H/I had a better effect on African Americans than on whites suggests skewed research. The FDA's conclusion was not based on conclusive evidence that BiDil had a unique level of efficacy for African Americans, as opposed to other racial ethnic groups. The FDA did not consider earlier H/I trials a sufficient basis for the drug's approval. Ironically, the FDA conducted research as a "good case" for African American heart failure research.

The purpose of clinical research is to assess all likely combinations of groups to determine where significant differences are located. Clinical research uses clinical trial processes to examine group comparisons. The comparison process used in the BiDil clinical trials was one of post hoc comparison. Post hoc groups are broken into three or more groups called subgroups. Subgroups are used to compare research findings, which was not the case with BiDil. Dr. Kirsten Bibbins-Domingo, endowed chair in medicine and professor of medicine and of epidemiology and biostatistics at the University of California, San Francisco (UCSF) and Dr. Alicia Fernandez, Professor of Clinical Medicine at UCSF, assert, "In general, post hoc subgroup analyses should be interpreted with caution and should be used primarily for generating hypothesis- not for determining policy, which appears to be the case here."[26] Gathering a sufficient number of participants for each subgroup is rare, which makes research difficult to satisfy sample sizes needed for accurate evaluations. Multiple post hoc subgroup analyses increase the risk of generating statistically significant and random group differences. Multiple subgroups can affect missing differences in data. Post hoc subgroups analyses are not a part of the original trial design.

Patients in subgroups are randomly allocated to intervention and control groups. Race and medicine expert Jonathan Kahn states, "The post hoc subgroup analyses of V-HeFT I and II suffer from the same potential problems as those faced by all post hoc subgroup analyses of randomized controlled trials: a loss of statistical power and the potential for covariate imbalances."[27] The data from BiDil's clinical trials was based on unclear post hoc data. The FDA's denial to Medco was evidence that Medco and Cohn's use of post hoc subgroups had vague and non-efficacious data.

NitroMed's clinical trials omitted mortality rates of senior citizens who have heart failure. NitroMed's age-focused interpretation obscures BiDil's data being effective in African Americans. In clinical trials, the misinterpretation and omission of data does not produce legitimate results. NitroMed used data from the 1981 National Center for Health Statistics, which described a black-to-white ratio of heart failure mortality (2:1).[28] In 1995, the Centers for Disease Control (CDC) stated patients 65 and older, with mortality rates from heart failure nearly equal for blacks and whites (a 1.1:1 ratio), were not included in NitroMed's data.[29] Ninety four percent of all heart failure mortality occurs over 65 years old. NitroMed had a distorted focus on data concentrating only on "patients aged from 45 to 64 years, thus boosting the black to white differential."[30] The interpretation of data suggests BiDil's effectiveness on African Americans resulted in the African Americans studied were prone to die from heart disease at a younger age.

African American subjects were the only trial group enrolled in the A-HeFT trial study. The absence of other racial populations in A-HeFT trial indicate BiDil should not have been presented and approved as a legitimate claim of differential efficacy based on race. By contrast, there were numerous drugs being tested in white populations, but no urgency to call these "Caucasian" or "European American" drugs. NitroMed was not being consistent in their vision of race-based medicine. Drugs being tested in all races would be attributed to specific races. Yet, race-based medicine was attributed only to Blacks or African Americans, which ignores other "racial" illnesses in other groups like Tay Sachs in Jews and Cystic Fibrosis in whites. NitroMed's concentration of African Americans suggests a financial attempt to capitalize on a specific racial group.

Race as Biocapital

NitroMed's approval, trials, and construction of BiDil illustrates biocapitalistic motives. The notion of biocapital is, "the circuits of land, labor, and value (in a classic Marxian sense) that are inhabited by biotechnology innovation and drug development; on the other hand, as the increasingly constitutive fact of biopolitics in processes of global capitalism."[31] In other words, biocapital is the merging of multiple modern systems of capitalism with developing sciences and technologies in life sciences (i.e. zoology, botany, microbiology, biology, biochemistry and physiology). In relation to BiDil, the biocapital element in this equation is race. NitroMed's role in biocapital creates alienation and expropriation that has been constructed on a notion of race, to express an innovative technique for pharmacology and biotechnology. Similar to commercial capitalism, race conjoined with biocapitalism is speculative— based on conjecture rather than knowledge. Race as biocapital influences medicalization and biomedicalization in racial groups.

Congestive heart failure produces 400,000–700,000 new cases per year with 750,000 African Americans out of 5 million Americans already affected, an estimate profit of $40 billion dollars annually.[32] NitroMed did not want inclusive participation of racial groups to happen because the non-racial patent will expire in 2007, but the African American race-specific patent will expire in 2020, which will give "NitroMed an additional 13 years of market monopoly protection"[33] compared to only two years for the non-race-based patent. NitroMed had better financial incentive marketing BiDil as an African American tailored medicine, which denotes racial targeting as their sales approach.

In 2005, it could take up to fifteen years to bring a drug to market costing an estimated price between $700 and $900 million and around $1.2 billion in 2010.[34] Yet, NitroMed cheated the drug development process. NitroMed only paid $43 million and brought BiDil to the market in five years by exploiting its race-based advantage.[35] A very unorthodox process for a drug which main ingredients H/I had been used as a non-racial "off label" prescription since the 1980s. The FDA's "off label" description states,

The drug label of FDA-approved drugs gives information about the drug, including the approved doses and how it's to be given to treat the medical condition for which it was approved. When a drug is used in a way that is different from that described in the FDA-approved drug label, it is said to be an "off-label" use. This can mean that the drug is:

- Used for a different disease or medical condition.
- Given in a different way (such as by a different route).
- Given in a different dose.

For example, when a chemotherapy drug is approved for treating one type of cancer, but is used to treat a different cancer, it is off-label use. Off-label is also called "non-approved" or "unapproved" use of a drug. New uses for these drugs may have been found, and often medical evidence supports the new use. But the makers of the drugs have not put them through the formal, lengthy, and often costly studies required by FDA to officially approve the drug for new uses.[36]

The "off label" H/I combination was so effective in the general population that the AHA endorsed it as an adequate treatment of heart failure for over fifteen years.

The "off label" H/I combination was a cheaper alternative for patients of all races that had heart failure issues, but did not have the financial means to obtain a prescription. African Americans are one of the main groups struggling economically. The average black household has less than one-tenth of the wealth of a typical white household[37] and the average white household has 16 times the wealth of the average black household.[38] NitroMed asserted the reason they made BiDil was to close the health disparity gap for African Americans dealing with heart failure.[39] It was logical and consistent with their claim to make BiDil affordable to such a disenfranchised group. Unfortunately, NitroMed's biocapitalistic motive superseded their pseudo-health equity initiative and focused on market-based goals.

NitroMed speculated the perceived innovation of BiDil will bring in a substantial amount of money. As Sunder states, "Biocaptial is the articulation of a technoscientific regime … over determined by the market."[40] Life sciences expedite the production of cutting edge technologies and therapeutic interventions. The results of such innovative technologies and interventions are ambiguous in nature. Regardless of the knowledge of these innovations, the market inputs the value of proposed technologies and interventions with intent to calculate their value and return on investments. NitroMed is a key example of the biocapitalistic process expediting the process of BiDil, which caused huge speculation in the stock market.

In 2004, a week after the A-HeFT trial completion, NitroMed's stock tripled from $6.90 per share to over $21 per share. In 2005, NitroMed stock went up to $29 per share after FDA approval. On June 27th, four days after BiDil's FDA approval, NitroMed set the cost to BiDil at $1.80 per pill, with a standard dose of six pills per day, totaling $10.80 per day.[41] BiDil cost three times more than Coreg (beta-blocker) $3.56 per day and seven times more than the $0.25 cents per pill "off label" H/I combination. BiDil's financial gain for NitroMed was set. NitroMed's next step was to appeal to the African American community through key partnerships.

NitroMed's key partnerships were with ABC, the National Minority Health Month Foundation (NMHMF), and U.S. Representative Donna Christensen (D-Virgin Islands). Before the FDA approval meeting of BiDil, the NMHMF held a joint press conference with prominent African American public health groups like the Alliance of Minority Medical Associations, the ABC, the International Society on Hypertension in Blacks, the National Association for the Advancement of Colored People (NAACP), and the National Medical Association urging the FDA to approve BiDil.[42] Specifically, the National Medical Association supported BiDil.[43] These groups argued that BiDil finally brought personalized medicine to the African American community. In contrast, not all African American health organizations were quick to jump on the BiDil band wagon.

The Alliance of the Minority Medical Associations' President Randall W. Maxey stated, "The assertion that this is a race drug is misguided."[44] Maxey strongly urged the FDA not to approve BiDil. One would think that the massive contradictions, uncertainties, and inconsistencies of BiDil's clinical process would influence key groups in African American public health to reject BiDil. Unfortunately, there emerged a conflict of interest. NitroMed knew their success would not be legitimate without the backing of key players in the African American public health community. NitroMed could not offer sound clinical data, but they could offer compensation to promote their product. NitroMed contributed $200,000 to the ABC, $14,000 to U.S. Representative Christensen, and an unrestricted educational grant to the NMHMF.[45] In support of NitroMed, Congresswoman Christensen said, "BiDil can save thousands of lives and reduce untold suffering for African American heart failure patients and their families."[46] Also, NitroMed gave the NAACP $1.5 million dollars.[47] The African American public health groups endorsements and BiDil's "innovation" to alleviate health disparities in communities of color (fueled by biocapital anticipations) was enough for BiDil's approval. Yet, ironically, a pill exclusively made for African Americans was too expensive for the group it was supposed to benefit.

A year after BiDil's release in the stock market, its stock value fell from $27.00 per share to $2.50 per share.[48] BiDil's lack of financial credibility is not surprising. When marketing a prescription product to the consumer-patient the two important factors are efficacy and affordability, which BiDil provided neither. The Veterans Health Administration (VHA) denied Tier 2 status to BiDil and criticized its cost effectiveness asserting, "The annual cost of BiDil would range from $1382 to $2765 per patient, while the annual cost of comparable generics would range from $45 to $63 per patient."[49] The VHA's evaluation of BiDil led them to conclude lower priced generics would save hospitals more money compared to using BiDil. Consequently, the entire ABC group did not recommend BiDil. Dr. Charles Curry, Head Cardiologist at Howard University and founding member of ABC, criticized BiDil's cost and wanted "practical doctors using generics instead."[50] ABC realized that the cost of BiDil did not make practical financial sense. The socially incompetent cost projection of BiDil led to its financial failing. Furthermore, the pricing of BiDil did not encourage physicians to prescribe it to their patients.

Most of the time physicians have their patients' best interests at heart. Many physicians were not comfortable integrating BiDil within their practices for three reasons: price, compliance, and veracity (truthfulness or truth-telling). In a study by the *Journal of General Internal Medicine*, "Physicians overwhelmingly voiced concern that commercial considerations shaped the development of BiDil and expressed dismay at what they perceived to be the primary aim of race-specific pharmaceutical trials, namely to get physicians' attention for marketing purposes."[51] NitroMed's reimbursement incentives was not favored by many doctors. It was not practical to use BiDil when other affordable options were available for their patients. Also, BiDil's regiment of consumption three times per day compromises the physician's responsibility for beneficence (doing good) and nonmaleficence (doing no harm) if the patient is already taking other drugs. BiDil may create issues of compliance in physicians' medical practices by fatal drug reactions that can produce unwanted comorbidities.

Physicians should value their patients trust. In BiDil's case, physicians should be even more sensitive to African Americans because of the group's egregious American medical history. Incorporating BiDil into the medical practice is a step backward because it medically "pimps" the African American community by doctors prescribing it. NitroMed's poor marketing and lack of physician support resulted in an unsuccessful attempt for race-based medicine. In 2009, Deerfield Capital acquired NitroMed for $36 million and planned to develop a more potent form of BiDil that can be taken once a day compared to three times a day and NicOx S.A. purchased NitroMed's unlicensed patents covering nitric oxide-donating compounds.[52] In 2012, Deerfield Capital Management sold the rights to BiDil to Arbor Pharmaceuticals, Inc. of Atlanta, Georgia.[53] Despite BiDil's unscientific prowess and reputation, Arbor Pharmaceuticals is capitalizing from BiDil and are "planning to do further research to try to predict more accurately which patients are most likely to respond to the treatment."[54] BiDil is still going strong in the drug market exploiting misunderstandings of race and disease.

NitroMed's construction of BiDil regurgitated the eugenic idea that race is a proxy for disease. As Johnathan Kahn profoundly asserts, "NitroMed put a 'black face' on BiDil as it went before the FDA for race-specific approval."[55] NitroMed medicalized race and it is attributing the pathology of heart failure to African Americans, which is historically and scientifically false. The biocapitalistic use of BiDil has medicalized and biomedicalized race in the twenty-first century.

Race: Medicalization and Biomedicalization

The FDA's second justification for approving BiDil was an ethical concern concerning racial difference. The FDA asserted, "Not understanding the reasons for the difference in treatment effect by race did not justify withholding the treatment from those who could benefit from it."[56] The FDA believed withholding BiDil from those who might benefit was not necessary and irresponsible. The FDA did not wait for a full understanding of how the drug worked. The FDA was irresponsible in expediting the drug when they had neither a clear understanding of its risks nor its benefits. Responsible pharmaceutical research requires time to properly assess the risks and benefits within a population, especially dealing with the complexities of race and socioeconomics. In regard to BiDil, the African American population should not be the victim of hurried research practices.

The FDA's undeveloped allegation that BiDil is a race-based drug while simultaneously stating they lack the full understanding of how the drug works exhibits poor science and weak judgment. The FDA's urgency to get BiDil in the drug market was internally induced and created the illusion that BiDil was a miracle pill for African Americans with heart issues. The FDA's statement is disingenuous and raises concern about FDA's upholding of the 1906 Food and Drug Act on drug approval and the 1962 Amendments.

The Food and Drug Act established precedent for regulation of medication by enforcing medicine, safety, efficacy, and prosecuted false drug claims. The Food and Drug Act, "Prevented the manufacture, sale, or transportation of misbranded, poisonous, or deleterious drugs and medicines."[57] The Act had unclear guidelines for compliance, which was mediated by the FFDC Act and the 1962 Amendments. The FFDC Act, "provided consumer protection by requiring scientific proof of the safety of new products, regulating therapeutic devices, making the prosecution of false drug claims easier, and raising the penalty of violators."[58] The 1962 Amendments set the precedence for drug efficacy and required:

> That adverse reactions of drugs be reported to the Food and Drug Administration, that risks and benefits of drugs accompany medical journal advertisements of drugs, *and that the effectiveness, as well as the safety, of a drug be proven before it is marketed.* (emphasis added)[59]

The FDA's approval of BiDil shows medicalization's effect on compliance regarding consumer protection and efficacy.

In 1972, Irving Zola framed the concept of medicalization as a precursor of the growing dominance of medicine's influence in jurisdiction, authority, and practice in society.[60] Prescribed medications for most of the twentieth century was used as a secondary option for the patient's therapeutic intervention. However, there was a huge shift beginning in the 1980s.

The rise of 'Direct-to-consumer' (DTC) marketing brought a new level of awareness about medical interventions to the American consumer, but the marketing was limited. Pharmaceutical companies could only place drug advertisements in popular magazines and newspapers. DTC marketing on drugs intensified in the 1990s with the passing of the Food and Drug Administration Modernization Act of 1997 which "loosened the restrictions placed on the kind of information that pharmaceutical companies could share with physicians regarding 'off label' uses of their drugs."[61] The Act influenced the approval of Paxil (paroxetine hydrochloride) for the treatment of depression with Prozac and other drugs (SSRIs) to follow. "Medicalization" quickly became dominant in mainstream American culture.

Medicalization is the process by which nonmedical issues become interpreted, defined, and treated as medical problems, and are then labelled as a certain illness or disorder. Medicalization simply means "to make medical."[62] Regular life events like menstruation, birth control, infertility, impotency, childbirth, menopause, aging, and death are now medicalized. As a result, patients are transformed into con sumers and are less tolerant dealing with the symptoms of life events (i.e. Viagra for men and women). Instead of the patients going through longer processes of healing, medicalization produced a "microwave" mentality in patients. Patients have an uncomfortable symptom. The therapeutic intervention was simply pop a pill or injection that will alleviate the symptom(s) quickly. A recent example of medicalization is the drug injection called Kybella (deoxycholic acid) made by Kythera Biopharmaceuticals in Westlake Village, California, which dissolves chin fat (double chin).[63] Medicalization promoted the prescription drug from a secondary medical intervention to a primary means in clinical practice, which enmeshed the pharmaceutical companies and patients in a markedly co-dependent relationship.

Medicalization changed the paternal model of doctoring. Patients became consumers and empowered to seek out medical interventions and services they desired with or without the doctor's approval. The traditional patient-physician power dynamics changed because if your doctor does not agree with you taking a prescription of personal interest or does not want to undergo a procedure, you can find a doctor that will comply with your desires. Medicalization engages life itself through the pursuit of enhancements to alleviate individuals' physiological inconsistencies and anxieties through medical forms of interventions.

The FDA's Modernization Act of 1997 opened the "Pandora's Box" of drug and medical marketing. Medicalization has created an oversaturation of drugs in the market, which has in turn affected the non-maleficence of the patient. According to the *Journal of the American Medical Association* March 2015 article, drug overdose deaths (by opiate pain and other medications) have been rising since the early 1990s and is the leading cause of injury death in the United States.[64] Due to the overwhelming access of drugs, the risks are greater compared to ten or fifteen years ago and side effects caused by medication generate countless risks. Regardless of the rise of alternative and homeopathic medicine, medicalization has ingrained a culture of medication as the main form of therapeutic intervention.

Medicalization's fallacy narrowly focuses on the source of the problem in the individual rather than including the social environment and calls for medical interventions not social solutions. Also, medicalization has its limitations because medical phenomena are intangible. For example, masturbation, hysteria, homosexuality, and drinking coffee[65] were deemed as medical issues, but views changed overtime. Likewise, race is a fluid concept that changes overtime. The approval of BiDil re-medicalized race within medicine through revived unorthodox eugenic ideologies in the FDA's approval meeting on BiDil.

As discussed, the racial research component of BiDil did come from John Cohn, but the racial medical language came from Robert Nissen, chair of the FDA Advisory Committee. After the FDA reviewed BiDil, Nissen asserted, "We're using self-identified race as a surrogate for genetic markers. It is very unusual; it is precedent-setting... But it is the case that we are moving forward to genome-based medicine. It's going to happen."[66] Nissen ignored the overwhelming data inconsistencies of the V-HeFT and A-HeFT trials and focused on racial difference as the only justification for BiDil's approval.

Nissen erroneously compared heart failure to orphan disease. Orphan disease consists of diseases like Hamburger disease, Lou Gehrig's disease, Job syndrome, cystic fibrosis, gigantism (acromegaly) and Tourette's syndrome. Orphan disease effects less than 200,000 people compared to 750,000 African Americans who suffered from heart failure in the United States.[67] Nissen's sample sizes were inconsistent because one cannot compare a disease that affects a general population group (Orphan Disease) to a racial group (Heart Failure). There is no scientific basis to use such an example as rationale and justification to approve BiDil.

Similar to FHS, BiDil's objectives were revised after data collections. Also, Nissen's interpretations skewed information to reflect a preferred result, which in BiDil's case was race.[68] As Jonathan Kahn states, "It was race itself that he connected to disease, people suffering from "African-American-ness' deserved the same special consideration as those suffering from an orphan disease."[69] Nissen's assertion reifies race as a biological truth that supersedes statistics, which led to the FDA's justification that race is a proxy for disease. Furthermore, the FDA biomedicalized (social processes are assigned meaning) race by approving BiDil as a form of enhancing personalized medicine for African Americans.

Biomedicalization practices, "emphasize transformations of such medical phenomena and of bodies, largely through sooner-rather-than-later technoscientific interventions not only for treatment, but also increasingly for enhancement."[70] Technoscience produce identity through applying science and technology to our bodies. Technoscience creates identities and labels exemplified in BiDil's case two ways. It imposes new mandates and performances that become incorporated into one's sense of self and creates new categories of health related identities and redefines old ones.[71]

Biomedicalization courts fatalism to create a mindset of vulnerability centered on risk factors and self-surveillance. Risk factors and self-surveillance are components of the medical gaze, which is the dehumanizing medical separation of the patient's body and personhood. Risk factors and self-surveillance construct the spaces, technologies, discourses, and processes of biomedicalization. These social constructions inject interventions around the risk and chronic diseases. Symptoms are obsolete due to,

The 'problematization of the normal' and the rise of what Armstrong (1995) calls 'surveillance medicine,' everyone is implicated in the process of being ill. Both individually and collectively, we inhabit tenuous and liminal spaces between illness and health, leading to the emergence of the 'worried well,' rendering us ready subjects for health-related discourses, commodities, services, procedures, and technologies.[72]

Similarly, race-based medicine affects minority communities' overall understandings of health through communicating false notions that external traits of minorities contribute to the cause of disease.

Race, understood to generalize a group of people who have similar physical and genetically coded traits, should therefore not be used to determine the development of drugs. There are many causes of disease like poor nutrition, lack of exercise, poor hygiene, heredity, and environmental factors. Race-based medicine accentuates a false fatalistic ideology that one's personal health habits are not significant for disease prevention compared to one's external racial traits.

NitroMed's implications through the biomedicalization of risk factors and self-surveillance related to BiDil recreated the eugenic stratification of racial bodies as biologically different. Such markers impose sociobiological and sociocultural perceptions that rationalize, "'different' kinds of bodies and the ways in which individuals so marked think about themselves and their health."[73] NitroMed's racial construction of BiDil was to project a familiar urgent fatalism to African Americans that have heart failure. The premise was that you are black, you are different, so take this drug that was specifically made for "people like you." Consequently, race and biomedicalization intersect with geneticization. Geneticization is a social process and genetic form of medicalization that centers genes as the core of interpreting meaning and genetic findings supersede historical sociological explanations.[74]

Genetics and Race

The FDA's third justification for approving BiDil is, "Regulatory and other concerns associated with drug approval for narrow patient populations did not justify withholding BiDil from those who could benefit from it."[75] The FDA's problematic justification naively overlooks the stigmatization of African Americans' heart failure. Stigmatization is the label or mark of disgrace toward a person or a group. The FDA approving BiDil stigmatizes African Americans by attributing and associating heart failure and unhealthy behavioral traits with African Americans. The perception of race-based medicine misconstrues the distinctions of race, ancestry and genetics by promoting assumptions that race alone is the only marker of disease. Clinical research of minorities needs to establish a precedent, Robert Temple and Norman L. Stockbridge asserts where, "evidence of a genetic basis for a racial distinction must clearly be shown before a race-specific approval, even in the face of compelling benefit in one race."[76] The FDA does not recognize the stigmatizing of race as a concern. Cultural competency in research and patient care is a fundamental necessity, which the FDA's approval of BiDil disregards.

Since 1950, the United Nations Educational, Scientific & Cultural Organization (UNESCO), the American Association of Physical Anthropologists, the International Union of Anthropological & Ethnological Sciences, the American Sociological Association, and the American Anthropological Association all agreed that race is not a proxy for biological explanations and difference.[77] Yet, the concept of race as an explanation for disease is still infiltrating science and medicine in the twenty first century.

The previously named institutions have indeed contributed to great progress on how we should view race in science and medicine. However, their bold statements do not erase the ingrained societal effects of racial ideologies in American society. Mentioned in Chapter 1, The United States Office of Management and Budget (OMB) constructed racial and ethnic categories used to collect, organize, and analyze the country's demographic data. Such information is collected through the census forms filled out periodically. OMB changed racial categories at least ten times since its inception in 1800.[78] For example, the first US Census listed,

Free White Male, Free White Female, Other Free Person, and Slave. During the nineteenth century, additional categories that fell in and out of use included Free Colored Person, Black, Mulatto, Quadroon, Octoroon, Indian, Chinese, and Japanese. The twentieth century saw a new proliferation of categories including Hindu, Korean, and Negro.[79]

On May 12, 1977, the OMB's Statistical Policy Directive No. 15, Race and Ethnic Standards for Federal Statistics and Administrative Reporting was produced to provide,

> Standard classifications for record keeping, collection, and presentation of data on race and ethnicity in Federal program administrative reporting and statistical activities. These classifications should not be interpreted as being scientific or anthropological in nature, nor should they be viewed as determinants of eligibility for participation in any Federal program. They have been developed in response to needs expressed by both the executive branch and the Congress to provide for the collection and use of compatible, nonduplicated, exchangeable racial and ethnic data by Federal agencies.[80]

After many changes, this process of taxonomy (classification) led to the categories of race and ethnicity we know today like: American Indian or Alaska Native, Asian, Black or African American, Native Hawaiian or Other Pacific Islander, with Hispanic or Latino and Not Hispanic or Latino as the two categories for ethnicity.[81] The OMB's categories are used on the local, state, and federal levels for research, data, and practice, which are used for public health issues and biomedical research.

The United States Patent and Trademark Office (PTO) has powerful influence through federal officials controlling the use of race into biomedicine. The PTO's decisions produce constructed racial categories used for the U.S. Census. The racial categories are used as a means of biological research that support the appropriation of race and biology in biomedicine. In fact, genetic research has rapidly grown since the completion of the Human Genome Project (HGP) in the early 2000s. The HGP was an international research effort to sequence and map all the genes of humanity, also known as the genome. The mass amount of data and knowledge obtained was tremendous. Such knowledge needs to be collected, stored, and classified as genetic information. The OMB and PTO racial categories are used in international biobanks. Hence, international federal governments sponsored data banks to maintain genetic data for biomedical researchers.

The databanks and databases are the National Institute of General Medical Sciences (NIGMS) under the Department of Coriell Human Genetic Variation Collections, the DNA Polymorphism Discovery Resource (PDR), the database of single-nucleotide polymorphisms (dbSNP database), the Haplotype Map Project (IHMP or HapMap), the National Center for Biotechnology Information (NCBI or GenBank), the DNA DataBank of Japan (DDBJ), and the European Molecular Biology Laboratory (EMBL).[82] These databases have unprecedented power in affecting how genetic information is used. Researchers use these databases to organize racial categories, genetic information, and apply genetic data by race classification. For example, the PDR's chief scientists, who were from the HGP, created race-based sample sets by federal race classification.[83]

Biobanks romanticized race with biomedicalization using classification. Classification is the assignment of organisms to groups within a system of categories distinguished by structure and origin. It implies class, order, and phylum (race, stock, or kind) of individuals and groups. Additionally, classification is defined by ethical choices that hold meaning and enable identification. However, classification inevitably excludes an individual or group as "the other" allowing different forms of hierarchy. Genetic classification profoundly describes the essence and character of a human being down to the cellular level. Genetic classification demonstrates power and danger because, "it involves biological categories that may be confused and conflated with race. Any resulting reification of social categories of race as biological constructs risks new forms of exclusion and stigma."[84]

The OMB, PTO and biobanks created an infrastructure of racialization which incorporated racialized labels for groups whose DNA samples they stored, resulting in the assertion of racial difference and genomics becoming the proxy for reading race.[85] Regardless of the international science community's statements that race is a myth, the biomedicalization of race became a priority. Researchers in science and medicine argued that race and equity are valid reasons to use race as a means for research. For example, Dr. Francis Collin said, "We need to try to understand what there is about genetic variation that is associated with disease risk, and how that correlates, in some very imperfect way, with self-identified race, and how we can use that correlation to reduce the risk of people getting sick."[86] Collins statement was the same rationale used in BiDil's 1050 "self-identified African-Americans" A-HeFT study.

The issue with "self-identification" of race is that it is based on subjectivity. Self-identification has no contextual validity, poor proxy of other people's perceptions, excludes people who cannot self-identify (i.e. multi-racial or bi-racial individuals), no use related to research questions on ancestry, and does not reflect the descent and ethnic origin of individuals.[87] Self-identification can be empowering and have elements of freedom, but it is a structural process predetermined by a set of classification recognized and enforced by the government (i.e. OMB and PTO).

In the American context, the precedent of racial self-identification was never set by individuals, but by the government over such individuals. However, American influences of self-identification, described in the book *Racisms: From the Crusades to the Twentieth Century*, came from Carl von Linnaeus and Johann Fredrich Blumenbach. Swedish botanist Carl von Linnaeus (1707–1778), known as the Father of Taxonomy, created the classification of skin color and first modern study of man. German anthropologist Johann Fredrich Blumenbach (1752–1840) included skin color, skull, and the physiognomy of man in 5 categories and coined the term Caucasian from the Caucasus Mountains.[88] Linnaeus and Blumenbach are important figures in the classification of racial groups.

Race, ethics, and self-determinism are influenced by social, political, and historical discourse controlled by the government. Eugenic history tells us that no one knows who they are until they are told by society and the society they are in is dictated by its government. A pertinent example is former Spokane, Washington, NAACP chapter president Rachel Dolezal. Dolezal created national headlines posing as an African American woman who was born a white woman.[89] She attributed to herself a black identity, but by an ingrained racial classification could not self-identify by societal terms. Self-identification does not have legitimate consensus among scientists and geneticists because it is not consistent with findings on the genetic level. For example, an interview with 30 geneticists used OMB categories of race in their studies and admitted the vagueness in classification and scientific inadequacy.[90]

Genetic variation is very complex within a group. Self-identification is used as a component in studying populations. Epidemiological research should be read through genetic ancestry and genome geography. Genetic ancestry alludes to the differentiations of populace. Geneticists use specific technologies to measure differences through genome-wide association studies (GWAS). GWAS researchers do not use race in their studies, but dispute their GWAS for disease associations require methods for accounting for population differences. The GWAS researchers developed tools that are more accurate than race groups accounting for population differences.[91] Genome geography is the tools and practices of human genetics, "bits of genomic sequence become associated with specific geographic locations, posited as the place of origin of people who possess these bits."[92]

Specifically, the tool used is EIGENSTRAT, a population genetics software technol-ogy. EIGENSTRAT is the type of technology that "moves from genetic similarity to genetic ancestry to genome geography."[93] GWAS focus on genetic markers called single nucleotide polymorphisms (SNPs). SNPs are markers of individuality and descent through parents. An SNP is a single base pair position in genomic DNA in "which two or more possible sequence alternatives (called 'variants') can occur. Researchers genotype each DNA sample, at each marker, to determine the pattern of variants in each case and con-trol individual. Geneticists estimate that there are about 10 million SNPs across the approximately 3 billion bases of the human genome, some of which lie within the approximately 20,000 to 25,000 genes."[94] This means that there are small genetic differences within humanity.

GWAS researchers use SNPs findings to determine which SNPs are related to disease. In human genetic variation studies, SNP vari-ants can vary across humans a SNP variant that is ordinary (or high in frequency) in one populace may be uncommon (or at low frequency) in another. It is possible the geneticist's SNPs findings were collected and labeled using racial or ethnic descriptors by group, but they declined to use such information. It is the ancestry and geographic location that should inform research for disease markers not race. It is important to understand geography and ancestry have a profound influence on physical attributes and disease of populations. A great example is the Pima Indians who, "have unusual susceptibility to non-insulin dependent diabetes mellitus, and the people of Gambia, in whom polymorphisms in the *NRAMP1* gene influence susceptibility to tuberculosis and the germ line *BRCA1* mutations that render Ashkenazi women susceptible to breast cancer resulting in generational inbreeding."[95]

One must consider an estimated 400,000 years of geographic scattering, genetic mixing and societal disorder among ancestors. Physicians, in the Intramural Research Program of the National Human Genome Research Institute and the NIH study, were skeptical about BiDil related to the issues of genetic mixing. There is not genetic proof that African Americans are genetically different than other racial groups. Consequently, Africans and African Americans are more genetically diverse among each other. The continent of Africa shows,

> DNA analysis of present day Africans reveals fourteen ancestral population clusters. DNA among African populations tends to be more variable and distinct than among populations from other continents. Even the term African American makes no sense genetically, as it implies unified population. The 20 percent average admixture of European alleles in African Americans, as well as the great genetic variation among different African populations, belies this biogeographic generalization.[96]

An allele is several forms of gene mutations that produce hereditary variation. It is evident certain alleles differ among certain populations.

Alleles are, "variant genes originated as mutations that proved advantageous under particular environmental conditions. In central and western Africa, for example, several independent mutations in the b-globin gene gave rise to different sickle hemoglobins, each with a distinct geographic distribution and phenotype."[97] These mutations multiplied throughout the populace as a form of defense against malaria. The mutation went to Iran, Greece, Turkey, Saudi Arabia, and other areas by migration and slavery. Another example is the FyO allele that is exclusively carried by West Africans and no other African or world population.[98] Human genomes are 3 billion base pairs spread across 23 chromosomes are 99.9% similar to one another with 0.1% difference (3 million pairs) with a smaller selection of 0.1% provide the raw material for locating the source of difference.[99] Diseases like sickle cell anemia and cystic fibrosis have nothing to do with race, but a reality of geography, ancestry and recessive mutations in specific genes. Hence, racialized medicine implies asymmetry in genetics.

Since ancestry and genome geography are better resources in discovering the origin and causes of disease, the reason researchers use uncritical notions of race in research should be challenged. The issue is researchers' biases about race in research, trials, and studies. GWAS and EIGENSTRAT tech-nologies present medical geneticists with an exact opportunity for data and research results. Rather than using the subjectivity of race or ethnic categories in the process of their research. This is possible by finding fresh ways, through GWAS and EIGENSTRAT tech-nologies, of doing genetic research on complex diseases. In the process of receiving samples of race or ethnic categories they, "need not be analyzed in those categorical terms."[100] EIGENSTRAT does not require the use of racial labels to describe research samples. Whoever decides to label and publish their analyses in terms of a racial category are doing so by their own discretion. As I mentioned earlier, the NIH Revitalization Act encourages the inclusion of women and racial minorities in clinical research. It also,

> mandates that practitioners in clin-ical and basic biomedical research receiving federal funding should *report* on the diver-sity of their research subjects according to racial and ethnic categories designated by the OMB. The regulations do *not require* either that the researchers must include members of all groups in their studies or that the researchers must *analyze* their samples using race categories. (emphasis added)[101]

GWAS technologies allows researchers to study complex diseases without the concept of race. It is the ethical duty of researchers to be self-aware of research bias and show an unprecedented approach to discontinue racial fatigue in biomedical research.

Race-based medicine is a step in the wrong direction because genetic relatedness overwhelmingly outweighs differences in human variation.

Race is dependent on one's cultural context, which makes race and genetics ambiguous and ripe for misappropriation and misinterpretation. For example, NitroMed used the term African American patient and the FDA used the term black patient.[102] Race as a proxy for disease not only creates uncertainty, but it can result in generalizations and stereotypes which can harm patients.

BiDil is harmful because it does not work in every African American or Black heart failure patient as the term "black heart drug" implies. Since African Americans or black individuals are genetically diverse, there cannot be a "one size fits all" drug. Adverse Drug Reactions (ADRs) to BiDil will inevitably be a dangerous reality because of the wide variability in its efficacy and toxicity. ADRs account for 100,000 patient deaths, 2.2 million injuries per year, and cost $174.4 billion dollars in the United States with a $101 billion dollar expense that could have been avoided.[103] BiDil's fast and cheap process ensures risk of ADRs for a population that is unethically simplified. The FDA's approval using race as a proxy for disease superseded scientific fact, which aggressively aided BiDil's race-based trend of clinical minstrelsy.

BiDil's race-based relatives were AstraZeneca's Iressa (gefitinib) and Alcon Laboratories' TRAVATAN. Iressa is a drug for non-small cell lung cancer (NSCLC), which causes 80% or 800,000 lung cancer deaths per year in Asia.[104] The "self-identified" East Asian participants were claimed to have an efficacious reaction to the drug approved by The Advisory Committee of the Japanese Ministry of Health. AstraZeneca's CEO Tom McKillop stated,

> As a responsible company, we have voluntarily withdrawn promotion of the product in the US market while we work with the FDA to ensure that Iressa is only taken by patients who are deriving from benefit. The dilemma we all face is that many people clearly benefit from Iressa, but it is currently difficult to determine exactly which are the patients most likely to do so. The advantages in patients of *Asian origin* demonstrated in our clinical trials and their experience to date has led the Advisory Committee of the Japanese Ministry of Health to recommend the continued availability of Iressa and has led to approval for the marketing of Iressa in China and other Asian markets. (emphasis added)[105]

Similar to NitroMed, AstraZeneca's findings did not have another racial control group to determine adequate racial efficacy of Iressa. McKillop's uncertainty illustrates an uncanny resemblance to the FDA's reaction to BiDil asserting race-based components without the proper clinical process to determine the proposed drug's efficacy. Another racialization of a condition was glaucoma.

TRAVATAN are eye drops that aid in the issue of glaucoma, which African Americans are at greater risk. African Americans are six to eight times at risk to develop glaucoma compared to the general population.[106] Glaucoma is an issue to the African American community, but glaucoma is not only a "black issue." Glaucoma is an issue for the public health for the general population. The race-based classification of conditions or diseases creates inaccurate scientific perceptions of different types of groups. Race-based health differences are "biologic expressions of race relations,"[107] which are interpreted as real demographic issues that need to be resolved. The FDA justified their fourth reason for approving BiDil through the lens of equity and justice.

Health Inequity and Discrimination

The FDA's fourth justification for approving BiDil was to reduce social and demographic injustice and inequity. The FDA asserted that, "Race and other demographic characteristics have long been important to consider in analysis of trials and as a matter of equity and justice."[108] Effectiveness in therapeutics requires one to look at the entire social context of a group. Misunderstanding and ignorance of a group does not aid in proper alleviation of disease. Simply giving a group a pill does not instantly remove illnesses and diseases. Legitimate pharmacology and therapeutics engages with the group within their historical and social context, to better understand the source of the illness. A Pharmaceutical company expediting drugs as a quick fix is a lethargic solution and intensifies inequity instead of diminishing it. Race-based medicine continues health inequities by not focusing on discrimination, psychosocial stress and diet and nutrition as factors.

As studies have shown, minorities suffer from health inequities in the United States. In American medicine, "epidemiological data has reflected and reinforced scientific thinking about race for more than 200 years."[109] Epidemiological data shows an overwhelming amount of evidence of racial inequalities in morbidity and mortality, which African Americans rank the highest. For example, the age-adjusted death rate for African Americans was 30% higher than whites. Specifically, rates from hypertension, kidney disease, diabetes, hypertensive renal disease, and septicemia are twice as high in African Americans as in white Americans. In response to heart related issues, "Cardiovascular disease accounts for the largest share of black-white difference in mortality (34.0%), but there are substantial contributions from infections (21.1%), trauma (10.7%), diabetes (8.5%), renal disease (4.0%), and cancer (3.4%)."[110] These horrible statistics are a result of historical disregard of African Americans by the American medical system. For example, the discrimination behind the Tuskegee and Henrietta Lacks studies are disturbing historical events that African Americans have been victims of a medical system encapsulating them into discriminatory labels by the marker of race.

Discrimination is the treatment, consideration, and distinction of where a person or group belongs rather than on individual merit. Racism is the belief that all members of each race possess characteristics or abilities specific to that race, especially to distinguish it as inferior or superior to another race or races. Labels enforced on African American patients can produce negative assumptions and pre-conceived notions by the doctor. The consequence of labels puts a huge mental strain on black patients. This is an important factor in mental health in the black community. Negative factors that contribute to poor mental health outcomes include, "unfair treatment and social disadvantage as well as other social stressors, such as inadequate levels of social support, neuroticism, the occurrence of life events, and chronic role strain."[111] Labels create poor communication, which in turn worsens health disparities. A patient having a transparent relationship with their physician is more likely to have better health outcomes. In contrast, a patient feeling judged is more reluctant to discuss their health because they feel condemned by a false label attributed to them, which worsens health outcomes.

Race-based medicine does not reduce the consequences created by discrimination and racism. Discrimination imposes an unbearable amount of stress on African Americans. The history of racism in America has left African Americans in poor health for generations. Racism influences every facet of American society. For African Americans, racism contributes to health disparities. The psychosocial stress factor is significant in black health. Stress effects every element of one's being. The unchangeable marker of race becomes a constant stressor every day, "it reveals intricate relationships among the brain, immune system, autonomic nervous system, and the hypothalamic pituitary-adrenal (HPA) axis, as well as, the ways in which unhealthy environmental stimuli can "get under the skin" of individuals to cause negative health outcomes."[112] An individual experiencing a lifetime of racism (from birth to adulthood) has a higher risk of diabetes, stroke, and hypertension.

Anthropologist Chris Kuzawa explains discrimination and stress creates a vicious generational cycle. Kuzawa declares, "The immediate consequence of this intergenerational effect is a higher risk of adverse birth outcomes, but there is also a lingering effect into adulthood, as adult chronic diseases like heart disease and diabetes can be traced in part to prenatal and early life conditions. Thus, the cycle begins again."[113] A good example of this is comparing infants' birth weight for U.S.-born black women, African-born black women, and U.S.-born white women.

Regarding birth weight, African-born black women's babies were almost identical to U.S.-born white women's babies. However, the birth weight results negatively went down for U.S.-born black women. Interestingly, the benefit of African and Caribbean-born women decreased, in a single generation. The results show that, "The first generation of girls born in the United States to mothers of African descent grew up to have girls of their own with lower mean birth weights a trend that shifted the distribution toward that of U.S.-born black women."[114] This suggests discrimination has a significant impact on black birth rates. Socioeconomics and residential location affect black birth rates and other health and wellness factors. A drug based on race is not a health solution, but a distraction that ignores the greater issue of environmental racial discrimination that contributes to health inequity in communities of color.

Race-based medicine leaves the patient in a helpless state. The patient's disease is based on a racial classification out of one's control. Clinical focus should not be on race-based medicine, but on preventative means toward health disparities and enhancing social equity. There are many solutions that can alleviate health inequity and discrimination in minority communities. Two essential responses to health inequity are strengthening the physician-patient relationship through the physician's cultural competency, empathy and awareness with a keen focus on diet and nutrition.

Physician-Patient Relationship: Cultural Competency

Race-based medicine "normalizes" patient care. It makes assumptions about homogenous models of care within racial groups, which are inconsistent with the individuality of every patient regardless of race. The role of the physician is to recognize and address their lack of awareness and communicate clearly with patients. Physicians should not categorize patients by race. Categorization based on race and socioeconomics can bring expectations based on unproven stereotypes, labels, and assumptions. The best option for physicians is to humanize patient interaction. A physician's patient identification should not be the "5'10 black male weighs 200 pounds." Better identifiers would be "Jim, the engineer with a wife and three kids." Categorization detaches a physician, but personalization engages the physician with the patient's life.

Race-based medicine significantly affects the physician's cultural competency because research based on false assumptions about racial groups portrays minorities in an inaccurate way, which influences the physician's perception and way of practice. Historic experiences impact African Americans trust in medicine and the devaluating of black bodies is the foundation of western medical history. One key action doctors can take in improving relations with minority communities is recognizing minority patients' collective histories and make it an individual sacred act to value minority patients by expressing that value in the clinical practice and public health.

Physicians need to have a solid sense of cultural and self-awareness, because it impacts on decision quality. Quantitative errors account for only a small fraction of misdiagnoses and mistreatments. Most misdiagnoses and mistreatments are qualitative errors in thinking.[115] Interacting with the patient from an individual and personalized level helps to alleviate bias and stereotypes.

Race-based medicine gives physicians a facile means for diagnosing a patient based on external traits compared to assessing the patient's unique social status. A physician's most dangerous practice is allowing clinical statistics to supersede personal communication in patient care. When physicians focus on numbers to influence thinking, errors stemming from judgmentalism and normative thinking will arise. As a result, "a conscientious professional develops and follows an incorrect strategy. A physician committing this kind of error violates a norm of conduct, particularly by failing to discharge moral obligations conscientiously."[116] The development and progression of incorrect strategies and questionable modes of conduct can be a consequence of subconscious and unrealized biases or phobias by the physician and race based research.

Self-awareness cannot therefore be limited to personal cognition, but emphasis should be among the collective or group awareness among physicians and their support staffs. Physicians need to be aware and acknowledge the predispositions and socioeconomic inequities existing in minority groups. Physicians and their staff should thoroughly understand the community and the people they are serving.

Personal, cultural, and collective awareness among physicians are essential for effective communication. The physician-patient relationship should revolve around communication which is, "the fundamental instrument by which the physician-patient relationship is crafted and by which therapeutic goals are achieved."[117] The physician should not have biases, phobias, and preconceived notions toward patients. Assumptions should be eliminated. Doctors need to ask basic questions, feel comfortable in this process, and be respectful, empathic, and nonjudgmental. Communication is most effective when there is full openness between the doctor and patient.

Furthermore, the patient should not verbally express themselves solely by communicating the physical issue, but should have the opportunity to talk about their life. As a result, the patient is individualized instead of being categorized. Personal conversation between the patient and doctor lays a firm foundation to fight subconscious biases the physician has towards the patient. Communication connects the physician with the patient. The physician communicating and understanding the patient removes labels that are a result of race-based statistics. Such practices result in veracity, and create and encourage respect. Respect is a fundamental aspect of care, which "discerns the personhood of human beings as creatures able to persevere powerfully and creatively in their aims."[118] Respect shows the physician has compassion (active regard to another's welfare), and allows the physician to discern patient's judgments, decisions, fears, attachments, likes, and hates. The patient's personal sharing creates a foundation of trustworthiness and integrity.

Empathic Communication

The divide between patient and physician is a process of reconciliation that starts with an empathic relationship. Self-awareness opens the physician up to becoming empathetic. Empathic understanding is also central to the provision of all person-centered, relationship-based health care. This capacity for accurate and compassionate empathy is partly contingent on the subjective experiences of the observer the extent to, which he or she has experienced the emotions being imputed to the other.[119] In other words, empathy is the ability to understand another's experience, to communicate and confirm that understanding with the other person and to then act in a helpful manner. The physician, for example, who has not grieved cannot fully simulate (empathize with) a grieving patient although during the process of therapy the practitioner will learn more about the range of feelings and behaviors that may characterize this patient's state of mind.

The accuracy of this empathic process with patients is nevertheless often difficult for health professionals to attain. Communities undergoing rapid transition, disadvantaged, or challenged in health care delivery need culturally competent and empathetic physicians. Any lack of shared assumptions or values can result in demoralization and depersonalization of both the health care professional and the patient. Race-based medicine encourages assumptions by attributing a group to a disease. Specifically, African Americans being linked to heart disease, heart failure and high blood pressure. Such associations can make the patient feel they are a part of a general health problem they have no control over.

Lack of empathy and cultural competency can dehumanize the patient. It makes the patient feel inadequate, insignificant, and objective. Many of the criticisms of medical care voiced by minority patients refer to what they perceive as inadequate interpersonal and communication skills, rather than deficiencies in the technical or procedural aspects of their care. Research implies that explicit articulation of empathy and other altruistic behaviors may benefit both physician and patient.[120] Yet, oddly enough, empathy is articulated infrequently in most physician-patient relationships. Moments when emotions were expressed by the patients were often overlooked by the physicians. For example, approximately 200 such moments, termed empathetic opportunities, the oncologists responded 22% of the time, and with lung cancer patients the empathetic response was 11%.[121]

In a November 2015 *New York Times* article titled "Minorities Get Less Pain Treatment in E.R.," reports whites receive more pain treatment in emergency rooms compared to African-Americans and other minorities. The article was based out of the Center of Disease Control (CDC) four year study. The sample size was 6710 visits to 350 emergency rooms by patients eighteen and older with acute abdominal pain. Compared with non-Hispanic white people, non-Hispanic blacks and other minorities were 22–30% less likely to receive pain medication.[122] This study can convey the idea of black hardiness as a reason why African Americans are treated differently. Such beliefs are still prevalent in society, but I would not suggest this idea to be a legitimate proxy for physicians and their treatment of patients.

The *New York Times* article illustrated an issue explicitly a result of poor communication. As Dr. Adil H. Haider, the director of the Center for Surgery and Public Health at Brigham and Women's Hospital in Boston, said: "It may be that different people communicate differently with their providers. If we as providers could improve our ability to better communicate with patients so that we could provide more patient-centered care, we'll be making several steps toward reducing and hopefully eliminating these disparities."[123] Overall, the physician's interactions and understanding the patient's vulnerability was a very important element in patient care.

The explanation of physicians' lack of empathy, interpersonal skills, cultural competency and communication skills further confirms they have not received sufficient training to develop or enhance the necessary interpersonal and culturally competent skills for patient-centered care. Physicians who were trained dramatically improved on communicating with their patients. Controlled, randomized studies, conducted by Dr. Balint at the Tavistock Clinic, have confirmed and extended that physicians attending an 8 hour communication skills training course showed statistically significant improvements in empathic behaviors such as asking for patient's understanding and expectations, offering reassurance, setting an agenda for the medical visit, and eliciting the full spectrum of patients' concerns.[124] Physicians who had received training were able to recognize patients,' "psychosocial problems 50% of the time, compared with 37% for the control group of physicians who had not participated in the 8 hour course."[125]

Physician's Self Awareness

Race-based medicine obstructs physicians' training rather than improving it. Labeling and assumptions through race-based research can create lack of self-awareness, which produce malpractice situations. Malpractice is the negligence, misconduct, lack of ordinary skill, or breach of duty in the performance of a professional service that results in injury or loss.[126] Less studied, but now receiving greater attention, are measures of how the liability system affects clinical care. The pressing need to improve quality and efficiency in health care mandates any liability reform also be evaluated based on clinically relevant metrics. Evidence suggests one way to achieve quality is providers showing more empathy to patients.

Investigators at Jefferson Medical College in Philadelphia studied how medical outcomes of diabetics treated on an outpatient basis were affected by empathy, defined as "a predominately cognitive attribute that involves an understanding and an intention to help."[127] The investigators found that physicians with high empathy scores had patients with higher rates of favorable clinical outcomes than those with lower empathy scores. In contrast, race-based medicine already asserts an unfavorable prognosis and empathy toward the patient and determined the proper therapeutic approach is through pharmaceutical drugs.

In contrast to race-based medicine, clinical empathy and cultural competency are essential elements of quality care, and is associated with improved patient satisfaction and adherence to treatment as well as fewer malpractice complaints. Empathetic engagement in patient care can contribute to patient satisfaction, trust and compliance, researchers concluded in a recent issue of Academic Medicine.[128] The lead investigator on the empathy study and author of the textbook *Empathy in Patient Care* Mohammadreza Hojat, PhD asserted, "Malpractice claims against physicians are more likely when the physician fails to establish a trusting relationship with the patient," says. Hojat's findings underscore those of a 1997 study published in The *Journal of the American Medical Association*, which stated that, "Primary care physicians who used more statements of orientation (educating patients about what to expect and the flow of a visit), laughed and used humor more, and tended to use more facilitation (soliciting patient' opinions, checking understanding, and encouraging patients to talk) experienced less medical claims than those who were less engaged."[129]

Race-based medicine does not allow a patient to have opinions of prognosis because patient diagnosis is already pre-determined through race-based research. Patients do not have the option to express their opinion of the diagnosis. The patient's understanding of the disease is misinterpreted by the assumptions of race. For example, an African American heart failure patient associates disease to their race rather than personal responsibility of well-being (e.g. diet, exercise, and managing stress). Associating a personal ailment to one's race is dehumanizing. As a result, blacks and Hispanics are more comfortable with physicians of their own race to avoid stereotypes.

Stereotypes and categorizations enhance the perceptions of similarities within groups and differences between groups. Physicians interpret others by their own perceptions of stereotypes which influence expectations, inferences, and impressions. Theory and research on clinical decision making suggests ambiguities in the physician's understanding may result in health disparities which are results of a physician's belief that blacks are less likely to comply with treatment.[130] Such disturbing responses rejuvenate similar ideas of the non-complaint black slave, soldier and prisoner. Stereotypes are the consequences of the racist ideologies and oral traditions of American medicine and biology. It is a medical ritual handed down by the mechanism of a medical tradition that damages clinical care.

Due to socioeconomic dynamics of power, black patients typically have less time in the clinical practice with white doctors who are viewed as verbally assertive. Specifically, verbal assertion by a white doctor is interpreted "speaking down" to a minority patient showing superiority and antagonism. African American patients were four times more likely to believe they will experience racism in doctor's offices with 58% of Hispanics and 65% of blacks very or somewhat concerned with racism in medical practice with family members.[131] Also, 64% of blacks believe they receive lower quality of care, one-third of blacks experience racism in some part of their lifetime when seeking healthcare, and 95% of black report discrimination.[132]

The physician's cultural competency, empathy, and awareness are crucial elements in improving health inequity in the clinical practice. When minority patients trust their physicians and doctors correct unconscious bias, minority communities can improve their health outcomes. Another key element in alleviating health inequity and discrimination is health education and access to healthy foods. Poor access to healthy food is an important factor in health disparities.

Diet and Nutrition

In the early 1990s, Scotland, a resident of a public housing sector scheme used the term food desert for the first time. Since that time, researchers have used food desert for different meanings in research. Food deserts were defined as "urban areas with 10 or fewer stores and no stores with more than 20 employees."[133] Food deserts can be urban areas were individuals cannot by food due to income. Also, food deserts possess unhealthy type and quality of foods rather than the number of foods, type and size of food stores available to residents (i.e. farmers' markets/supermarkets vs. fast food chains). These definitions make it difficult to come up with a general agreement of what is an adequate definition of a food desert and what guidelines are required for identifying food deserts.

In the United States, food deserts are a health phenomenon. Many theories have been proposed on how food deserts came into existence. The first theory explains the expansion and closure of supermarkets, which hindered supermarket growth in urban/inner city areas, and stimulated the growth of large chain supermarkets in affluent suburban areas where consumers have better quality, variety and price for food options. In the suburbs, stores are more suitable for consumers having longer business hours and better parking options. These supermarkets have crippled the smaller, "mom and pop," neighborhood grocery stores competitive edge. Consequently, the neighborhood grocery stores are going out of business and individuals who want quality food will have to access it by a car or public transportation, which limits the geographical access to quality food. By this theory, an independent retailer asserts a food desert is "an area where high competition from the multiples [large chain supermarkets] has created a void."[134]

The second theory reflects on the demographics of urban areas between 1970 and 1988. Within this period, geographic and economic segregation grew when households of higher socioeconomic status moved from the inner-city to the suburbs. This reallocation cut the median income of urban areas and "forced nearly one-half of the supermarkets in the three largest U.S. cities (i.e. New York, Chicago, and Los Angeles in the 1970s and 1980s) to close."[135] As urban areas become more densely populated, supermarkets find urban areas unappealing due to the scarcity of real estate and zoning laws. It is very difficult for large supermarkets to find an adequate size of land, because properties are sold in smaller pieces, and since most individuals in urban areas occupy a lower socioeconomic status the monetary gain will not be in large chain supermarkets best interests.

Indeed, residents living in urban areas have their challenges obtaining healthy food. Research shows individuals living in rural communities encounter spatial disparity, because greater distances enhance one's inability to obtain essential goods and services. However, research on spatial distribution of food resources in rural communities is very scarce. There is a huge need for more research to be done regarding rural communities and its relation to food deserts. Nevertheless, let's focus on New York City and its relation to supermarket access in specific communities.

The Journal of Economic Geography did a study "to illustrate the effects on the measurement of disparities in food environments of adjusting for cross-neighborhood variation in vehicle ownership rates, public transit access, and impediments to pedestrian travel, such as crime and poor traffic safety."[136] The study used geographic information systems data of 2172 tracts from the 2000 census for New York City supermarkets, fruit and vegetable markets, and farmers' markets. The analysis used racial/ethnic and economic composition as categories. Specifically, the racial/ethnic and economic composition was broken down into five categories: majority (more than half) non-Hispanic white, majority non-Hispanic black, majority Hispanic, majority Asian or Pacific Islander, and a remaining group of census tracts which did not have any racial or ethnic group as a majority.

Additionally, the study compared 50% of foreign-born residents to those with 50% or less foreign-born population. The economic measurements were recorded by quartiles based on poverty rates, defined as the proportion of residents living below the federal poverty line.[137] The study used supermarkets data, from 2005, which categorized all grocery stores as supermarkets that were not termed as "convenience stores," had 17 or more employees, and had annual sales of $2 million. The studies result illustrated "New York City contains many densely settled neighborhoods that are characterized by mixed land use; in such neighborhoods, which are particularly prevalent in Manhattan and the innermost sections of Brooklyn, Queens, and the Bronx, the density of healthy food outlets is relatively high."[138]

Based on these results, the areas with the lowest access to healthy foods are in the outer edges of Bronx, Queens, Brooklyn, and in Staten Island. Since the average distance calculated was 800 meters, one needs to note that the distance of travel may not be adequate to confirm travel as a burden. The effects of smaller retailers, fruit and vegetable markets in relation to disparities by neighborhood race/ethnic, immigrant, or poverty had inconclusive measures regarding healthy food access.

Another interesting study by the *American Journal of Preventive Medicine* examined how urban food environments change over the course of one year. The study was based in Buffalo, NY. The data was from the 2000 U.S. Census, a 2010 listing of city supermarkets, 2011 government records and mapped location of urban farmers' markets.[139] The distances from block groups to supermarkets and farmers' markets were calculated. A 2011 written computer simulation examined the market closest to each block group for 52 weeks. The results show the average distance to supermarkets from block groups with poverty levels "in the top 10th percentile is greater than that across all block groups during winter and spring months."[140]

This study reflects that the wealthier block groups have greater access to supermarkets and farmers' markets compared to the poorer block groups, because "wealthier households have more economic resources and therefore attract farmers who perceive these regions as being areas with more demand."[141] During farmers' market season, low income neighborhoods have greater access to healthy food in warmer weather compared to colder weather, and low income areas with a higher frequency of poverty have a higher average distance to supermarkets and farmers' markets, than all block groups combined during the winter weeks. This can have huge influence on how food outreach programs are carried out. Poorer neighborhoods could be used as leverage in warmer weeks and wealthier households in the winter.

The NYC and Buffalo, NY studies show that access to healthy food is a complicated task depending on where you are from. Some areas may be less susceptible than others. The NYC study is an exception to geographic access to healthy food to low income households. According to the US Department of Agriculture (USDA) Economic Research Service (ERS) and the 2010 Census and supermarket data, "limited access to major food outlets such as grocery stores and supermarkets affects over 23.5 million people living in 6529 different Census tracts. 29.7 million people who lived in low income areas were over 1 mile from a supermarket."[142] The NYC analysis differed on access being an issue with healthy food, but it did assert, "The relationship between physical distance and travel burden is likely to depend on both individual/household and neighborhood characteristics."[143] Arguably, lower income households and neighborhoods can vary in physical access to food, but financial and geographical access creates huge challenges. Furthermore, the geographical and financial challenges low income households experience to obtain healthy food access is detrimental to these individuals health. These individuals lack of access to healthy foods results in poor nutrition.

Poor supermarket access creates discernable negative outcomes of residents consuming and being exposed to energy-dense food or "empty calorie" food available at convenience stores and fast-food restaurants. Research shows, "a diet filled with processed foods, frequently containing high contents of fat, sugar and sodium, often leading to poorer health outcomes compared to a diet high in complex carbohydrates and fiber."[144] The lack of supermarket access and poor nutrition are results of poverty. As the cost of healthy food continues to rise, barriers to healthy eating are created. People tend to make food choices based on what is available in their immediate neighborhood. This can produce problems since many low-income urban areas have a higher density of fast-food restaurants and corner stores that offer prepared foods compared to higher income areas.[145] For individuals in low income areas, it is more conducive to consume food that is cheap and local, rather than food that cost more at a farther distance.

Fruits and vegetables are vital to a healthy diet. The 2005 American Dietary Guidelines instructs 4.5 cups (9 servings) of fruits and vegetables daily, based on a 2000-calorie diet. Americans roughly consume 2.6 cups of fruits and vegetables.[146] Most Americans do not meet the 4.5 cup minimum, making the increase of fruit and vegetables intake an important goal for healthy eating interventions. In 2018, the food pyramid has been replaced by what should be on one's plate. One should make half the plate fruits and vegetables, focus on whole fruits, vary your veggies and half of your grains should be whole grains. Also, it is suggested to move to low-fat and fat-free milk or yogurt, vary one's protein routine, drink and eat less sodium, saturated fat, and added sugars.

Food environments influence a range of dietary health indicators including obesity rates, as well as the consumption of fruits, vegetables and low-fat dairy products. Failing to consume fruits and vegetables and other healthy foods daily can lead to a series of adverse health disparities, including obesity, diabetes, cancer, and cardiovascular diseases,[147] within low-income groups.

The Centers of Disease Control and Prevention (CDC) define health disparities as "preventable differences in the burden of disease, injury, violence, or opportunities to achieve optimal health that are experienced by socially disadvantaged populations."[148] The rise in obesity rates in the US has been a driving force of research into "obesogenic environments" (food environment–diet relationship). Studies assert food environments that have a lot of fast-food restaurants and few grocery stores were associated with higher odds of obesity among area residents.[149] Since food deserts create unhealthy communities, solutions need to be in place to sustain health equity and eradicate food deserts.

The first solution is creating initiatives to educate communities about health. Health literacy should start in low income communities. According to Judith C. Rodriguez, President of American Diabetes Association, "Only 12% of adults have proficient health literacy, as defined by the National Assessment of Adult Literacy (NAAL). In other words, nearly 9 in 10 adults may lack the skills needed to manage their own health and prevent disease. According to the NAAL, 14% of adults (30 million people) have below basic health literacy. These adults are more likely to report their health as poor (42%) and are more likely to lack health insurance (28%) than adults with proficient health literacy."[150] Policy makers, researchers and health professionals should work together and consider urban environments as entities were health education is a priority. By doing this, health education programs can improve health outcomes and produce cost-effective advancements in diets within low income communities.

More research in the unique dynamics of rural and urban food deserts is needed to better understand how food deserts are created and how they can be prevented. One innovative way to study rural and urban areas is through social media. In a study from *Applied Geography Journal*, food-related activities from social media Twitter, "tweets" provide an ideal method for measuring the exposure to the food environment in real time. The measure reflects food choices people make on twitter and where they decide to eat. The study compares "groups of Twitter users who shop in grocery stores to those who dine at fast food restaurants, we found that the prevalence of grocery stores that stock fresh produce within an individual's neighborhood may significantly influence him or her to make nutritious food choices."[151] Studies like this can be a great asset in understanding individual behaviors in how they chose food and what reasons are behind their dietary choices.

The second solution is improving food access. In the *American Journal of Preventive Medicine* study, Buffalo, NY had issues with low income households not having consistent access to healthy food through farmers' markets. Buffalo's solution was having farmers' markets accept purchases through the Women, Infants, and Children (WIC) and Seniors Farmers' Market Nutrition programs. This process can be the blueprint for other communities that are categorized as food deserts. Since location to supermarkets is a challenge, it is wise to bring the healthy food to the neighborhoods that need it the most.

Food deserts are making the most financially vulnerable around us ill. Poverty is a disease that negatively impacts the health of individuals. Furthermore, poverty prevents individuals from access to healthy foods through the distance of supermarkets. The lack of access to supermarkets leads to unhealthy eating habits, resulting in health disparities that can be prevented. Through health literacy and better access to healthy foods, food deserts can be eliminated and can aid in the elimination of health disparities.

Race-based medicine hinders a minority groups' self-awareness to make a conscience educated choice by turning their attention toward their physical traits and focusing on their race as a marker for disease. As a result, race-based medicine continues disinformation about race, its relation to disease and the genetic uniqueness of human beings. One should carefully evaluate the social and historical factors that affect the health of minority communities. Race-based medicine undermines the voice, participation, and interdependence of minorities by establishing false assumptions that race is the element for the origin of diseases and capitalizing on recurring eugenic ideologies. Such ideologies affect African Americans' understanding and language of personal health.

As discussed in Chapter 2, oral tradition has communal importance in the black community. It is a means where language depends on action or inaction. The fatalistic language of race-based medicine takes away the voice of the minority patient because inevitable illness purports a fixed epidemiological process. Physician's cultural competency, empathy, awareness and better nutrition are good suggestions for better health outcomes in minority communities. Furthermore, the use of black theology and the black church have given a voice for the minority community in situations when black voices have been quieted. Hence, black theology and the black church are versatile tools that can challenge race-based medicine.

The black church brings justice through health advocacy not allowing the health of oppressed groups to be ignored, responding to the poor socioenvironmental factors that contribute to minority groups' health inequity, and demanding the faulty solution of race-based medicine to be replaced with legitimate social solutions. Black theology is a tool to emphasize autonomy (freedom) in minority communities by encouraging the uniqueness and value of minority communities against the labels race-based medicine enforces. Chapter 4 will examine race in biblical literature, scripture as a tool for minority patient empowerment, and how faith communities' can play a significant role in health advocacy.

Notes

1. Pollock, Anne. *Medicating Race: Heart Disease and Durable Preoccupations with Difference*. Durham: Duke University Press, 2012, 31.
2. Aronowitz, Robert A. *Making Sense of Illness: Science, Society, and Disease*. Cambridge, UK: Cambridge University Press, 1998, 118.
3. Ibid., 55.
4. Pollock, *Medicating Race*, 54.
5. Aronowitz, *Making Sense of Illness*, 131.
6. Pollock, *Medicating Race*, 32.
7. Ibid.
8. Ibid., 28.
9. Ibid., 36–37.
10. Pollock, *Medicating Race*, 34.

11. Schwartz, Pamela Yew. "Why Is Neurasthenia Important in Asian Cultures?" *Western Journal of Medicine* 176, no. 4 (2002), 257–258.
12. Aronowitz, *Making Sense of Illness*, 119.
13. Ibid., 131.
14. Kahn, Jonathan. "Exploiting Race in Drug Development: BiDil's Interim Model of Pharmacogenomics." *Social Studies of Science* 38, no. 5 (October 2008), 738 (Sage Publications Ltd.).
15. Kahn, Jonathan. *Race in a Bottle: The Story of BiDil and Racialized Medicine in a Post-Genomic Age*. New York: Columbia University Press, 2013, 54.
16. Fuqua, Sonja R., et al. "Recruiting African-American Research Participation in the Jackson Heart Study: Methods, Response Rates, and Sample Description." *Ethnicity Disease* 15, no. 4, Suppl. 6 (2005), S6-18.
17. Briggs, Charles L. "Communicability, Racial Discourse, and Disease." *Annual Review of Anthropology* 34, no. 1 (2005), 280.
18. Fuqua, "Recruiting African-American Research Participation," S6-18.
19. Kahn, *Race in a Bottle*, 56.
20. Kahn, *Race in a Bottle*, 59.
21. Ibid.
22. Kahn, "Exploiting Race," 739.
23. Ibid.
24. Temple, Robert, and Norman L. Stockbridge. "BiDil for Heart Failure in Black Patients: The U.S. Food and Drug Administration Perspective." *Annals of Internal Medicine* 146, no. 1 (January 2, 2007), 57–59.
25. Ibid., 57.
26. Kahn, *Race in a Bottle*, 93.
27. Kahn, Jonathan D., et al. "Flaws in the U.S. Food and Drug Administration's Rationale for Supporting the Development and Approval of BiDil as a Treatment for Heart Failure Only in Black Patients." *Journal of Law, Medicine & Ethics* 36, no. 3 (Fall 2008), 450.
28. Kahn, *Race in a Bottle*, 72–78.
29. Ibid.
30. "Illuminating BiDil." *Nature Biotechnology* 23, no. 8 (August 2005), 903.
31. Sunder Rajan, Kaushik. *Biocapital: The Constitution of Postgenomic Life*. Durham: Duke University Press, 2006, 78.
32. Kahn, *Race in a Bottle*, 50.

33. Kahn, "Exploiting Race," 739.
34. Kahn, *Race in a Bottle*, 88.
35. Ibid., 92.
36. FDA. "Understanding Investigational Drugs and Off Label Use of Approved Drugs." Last modified June 24, 2015. http://www.fda.gov/ForPatients/Other/OffLabel/default.htm.
37. Luhby, Tami. "5 Disturbing Stats on Black-White Inequality." *CNN*. August 21, 2014. Accessed on July 18, 2015. http://money.cnn.com/2014/08/21/news/economy/black-white-inequality/.
38. Shin, Laura. "The Racial Wealth Gap: Why A Typical White Household Has 16 Times the Wealth of a Black One." *Forbes*, March 26, 2015. Accessed on July 18, 2015. http://www.forbes.com/sites/laurashin/2015/03/26/the-racial-wealth-gap-why-a-typical-white-household-has-16-times-the-wealth-of-a-black-one/.
39. Kahn, *Race in a Bottle*, 216.
40. Sunder, *Biocapital*, 111.
41. Kahn, *Race in a Bottle*, 103–104.
42. Kahn, *Race in a Bottle*, 101.
43. Briggs, "Communicability, Racial Discourse, and Disease," 281.
44. Kahn, *Race in a Bottle*, 101.
45. Ibid.
46. Inda, Jonathan Xavier. "For Blacks Only: Pharmaceuticals, Genetics, and the Racial Politics of Life." *Materiali Foucaultiani* I, no. 2 (2012), 108.
47. Bell, Susan E., and Anne E. Figert. *Reimagining (Bio)Medicalization, Pharmaceuticals and Genetics: Old Critiques and New Engagements.* Routledge: New York, 2015, 182.
48. Pollock, *Medicating Race*, 165.
49. Kahn, *Race in a Bottle*, 117.
50. Pollock, *Medicating Race*, 167.
51. Kahn, *Race in a Bottle*, 120.
52. Krimsky, Sheldon. "The Art of Medicine: The Short Life of a Race Drug." *Lancet* 379, no. 9811 (January 14, 2012), 115.
53. Hawkins-Taylor, Chamika, and Angeline M. Carlson. "Communication Strategies Must Be Tailored to a Medication's Targeted Population: Lessons from the Case of BiDil." *American Health & Drug Benefits* 6, no. 7 (2013), 408.
54. Downey, Laurence J. "BiDil: Alive and Kicking." *Lancet* 379, no. 9829 (May 19, 2012), 1876.
55. Kahn, *Race in a Bottle*, 102.

56. Temple, "BiDil for Heart Failure in Black Patients," 58–59.
57. Zarcadoolas, Christina, et al. *Advancing Health Literacy: A Framework for Understanding and Action*, 1st ed. San Francisco, CA: Jossey-Bass, (June 5, 2006), 26.
58. Ibid., 26–27.
59. Ibid.
60. Clarke, Adele. *Biomedicalization: Technoscience, Health, and Illness in the U.S.* Durham, NC: Duke University Press, 2010, 20.
61. Conrad, Peter. *The Medicalization of Society: On the Transformation of Human Conditions into Treatable Disorders.* Baltimore: Johns Hopkins University Press, 2007, 17.
62. Ibid., 4.
63. Food & Drug Administration. "FDA Approves Treatment for Fat Below the Chin." *FDA*, April 29. Accessed on April 29, 2015. http://www.fda.gov/NewsEvents/Newsroom/PressAnnouncements/ucm444978.htm.
64. Haffajee, R. L., A. B. Jena, and S. G. Weiner. "Mandatory Use of Prescription Drug Monitoring Programs." *JAMA—Journal of the American Medical Association* 313, no. 9 (March 3, 2015), 891–892.
65. LaMotte, Sandee. "Health Effects of Coffee: Where Do We Stand?" *CNN*, August 14, 2015. Accessed on August 16, 2015. http://www.cnn.com/2015/08/14/health/coffee-health/index.html.
66. Kahn, *Race in a Bottle*, 89.
67. Ibid., 98.
68. Shim, Janet K. *Heart-Sick: The Politics of Risk, Inequality, and Heart Disease.* New York and London: New York University Press, 2014, 55.
69. Kahn, *Race in a Bottle*, 98.
70. Clarke, *Biomedicalization*, 2.
71. Ibid., 81.
72. Ibid., 64.
73. Clarke, *Biomedicalization*, 220.
74. Bell, *Reimagining (Bio)Medicalization*, 176.
75. Temple, "BiDil for Heart Failure in Black Patients," 58–59.
76. Ibid., 61.
77. Bliss, Catherine. *Race Decoded: The Genomic Fight for Social Justice.* Stanford, CA: Stanford University Press, 2012, 3.
78. Wailoo, et al., *Genetics and the Unsettled Past*, 52.
79. Kahn, *Race in a Bottle*, 28.

80. CDC. "Statistical Policy Directive No. 15, Race and Ethnic Standards for Federal Statistics and Administrative Reporting." *CDC*, May 12, 1977. Accessed on August 20, 2015. http://wonder.cdc.gov/wonder/help/populations/bridged-race/directive15.html.

81. Kahn, *Race in a Bottle*, 28.

82. Ibid., 30.

83. Bell, *Reimagining (Bio)Medicalization*, 179.

84. Kahn, *Race in a Bottle*, 33.

85. Bell, *Reimagining (Bio)Medicalization*, 59.

86. Bell, *Reimagining (Bio)Medicalization*, 180.

87. Whitmarsh, et al., *What's the Use of Race?*, 128.

88. Bethencourt, Francisco. *Racisms: From the Crusades to the Twentieth Century*. Princeton: Princeton University Press, 2014, 250–253.

89. Johnson, Kirk, et al. "Rachel Dolezal, in Center of Storm, Is Defiant: 'I Identify as Black.'" *New York Times*, June 16, 2015. Accessed on July 7, 2015. http://www.nytimes.com/2015/06/17/us/rachel-dolezal-nbc-today-show.html.

90. Wailoo, et al., *Genetics and the Unsettled Past*, 52.

91. Fujimura, "Different Differences," 6.

92. Ibid., 7.

93. Ibid.

94. Ibid., 9.

95. Schwartz, Robert S. "Racial Profiling in Medical Research." *The New England Journal of Medicine* 344, no. 18 (May 3, 2001), 1392–1393.

96. Wailoo, et al., *Genetics and the Unsettled Past*, 59.

97. Schwartz, "Racial Profiling," 1393.

98. Wailoo, et al., *Genetics and the Unsettled Past*, 53.

99. Ibid., 16.

100. Fujimura, "Different Differences," 21.

101. Fujimura, "Different Differences," 21.

102. Kahn, *Race in a Bottle*, 10.

103. Wailoo, et al., *Genetics and the Unsettled Past*, 166–167.

104. Ibid., 176.

105. Ibid.

106. Rose, Nikolas S. *Politics of Life Itself: Biomedicine, Power, and Subjectivity in the Twenty-First Century*. Princeton: Princeton University Press, 2007, 181.

107. Kahn, *Race in a Bottle*, 6.

108. Temple, "BiDil for Heart Failure in Black Patients," 58–59.
109. Gravlee, Clarence C. "How Race Becomes Biology: Embodiment of Social Inequality." *American Journal of Physical Anthropology* 139, no. 1 (May 2009), 48.
110. Ibid.
111. Mays, Vickie M., et al. "Race, Race-Based Discrimination, and Health Outcomes Among African Americans." *Annual Review of Psychology* 58 (January 2007), 206.
112. Ibid., 205.
113. Gravlee, "How Race Becomes Biology," 52.
114. Ibid., 53.
115. White III, Augustus A. *Seeing Patients: Unconscious Bias in Health Care*. Cambridge: Harvard University Press, 2011, 204.
116. Beauchamp, Tom, and James Childress. *Principles of Biomedical Ethics*, 6th ed. Oxford: Oxford University Press, 2008, 34.
117. White, *Seeing Patients*, 199–200.
118. Stith, Richard. Toward Freedom from Value. *The Jurist* 38 (1978), 170.
119. Cox, John L. "Empathy, Identity and Engagement in Person-Centered Medicine: The Sociocultural Context." *Journal of Evaluation in Clinical Practice* 17, no. 2 (April 2011), 351.
120. Buckman, Robert, et al. "Empathic Responses in Clinical Practice: Intuition or Tuition?" *CMAJ: Canadian Medical Association Journal* 183, no. 5 (March 22, 2011), 569.
121. Ibid.
122. Bakalar, Nicholas. "Minorities Get Less Pain Treatment in E. R." *New York Times*. November 30, 2015. Accessed on December 2, 2015. http://well.blogs.nytimes.com/2015/11/30/minorities-get-less-pain-treatment-in-e-r/?ref=health&_r=0.
123. Ibid.
124. Neuwirth, Zeev E. "Physician Empathy—Should We Care?" *The Lancet* 350, no. 9078 (August 30, 1997), 606.
125. Neuwirth, "Physician Empathy," 606.
126. "Malpractice," *Encyclopedia Britannica*. Encyclopedia Britannica Inc., 2014. Web. November 10, 2014. http://www.britannica.com.ezproxy.drew.edu/EBchecked/topic/360514/malpractice.
127. McKnight, Whitney. *Infectious Disease News* 24, no. 6 (June 2011).
128. McKnight, *Infectious Disease News* 24, no. 6.

129. Ibid.
130. Smedley, Brian D., Adrienne Y. Stith, and Alan R. Nelson. *Unequal Treatment: Confronting Racial and Ethnic Disparities in Health Care.* Washington, DC: National Academy Press, 2003, 167, 173.
131. Ibid., 136.
132. Ibid.
133. Walker, Renee E., Christopher R. Keane, and Jessica G. Burke. "Disparities and Access to Healthy Food in the United States: A Review of Food Deserts Literature." *Health & Place* 16, no. 5 (September 2010), 876.
134. Walker, et al., "Disparities and Access to Healthy Food," 876.
135. Ibid., 877 (emphasis added).
136. Bader, Michael D. M., et al. "Disparities in Neighborhood Food Environments: Implications of Measurement Strategies." *Economic Geography* 86, no. 4 (October 2010), 409.
137. Ibid., 414.
138. Bader, et al., "Disparities in Neighborhood Food Environments," 417.
139. Widener, Michael J., Sara S. Metcalf, and Yaneer Bar-Yam. "Dynamic Urban Food Environments: A Temporal Analysis of Access to Healthy Foods." *American Journal of Preventive Medicine* 41, no. 4 (October 2011), 439.
140. Ibid., 440.
141. Widener, et al., "Dynamic Urban Food Environments," 439.
142. Sohi, Inderbir, Bethany A. Bell, Jihong Liu, Sarah E. Battersby, and Angela D. Liese. "Differences in Food Environment Perceptions and Spatial Attributes of Food Shopping Between Residents of Low and High Food Access Areas." *Journal of Nutrition Education and Behavior* 46, no. 4 (2014), 1.
143. Bader, et al., "Disparities in Neighborhood Food Environments," 412.
144. Walker, et al., "Disparities and Access to Healthy Food in the United States," 877.
145. Ibid.
146. Dean, Wesley R., and Joseph R. Sharkey. "Rural and Urban Differences in the Associations Between Characteristics of the Community Food Environment and Fruit and Vegetable Intake." *Journal of Nutrition Education & Behavior* 43, no. 6 (November 2011), 426.

147. Chen, Xiang, and Xining Yang. "Does Food Environment Influence Food Choices? A Geographical Analysis Through 'Tweets'." *Applied Geography* 51 (2014), 82.
148. CDC. *Community Health and Program Services (CHAPS): Health Disparities Among Racial/Ethnic Populations.* Atlanta: U.S. Department of Health and Human Services, 2008.
149. Sohi, et al., "Differences in Food Environment Perceptions," 1.
150. Rodriguez, Judith C. "Serving the Public: Health Literacy and Food Deserts." *Journal of the American Dietetic Association* 111 (January 2011), 14.
151. Chen, et al., "Does Food Environment Influence Food Choices," 82.

5

Black Theology and Reconciliation

So far, we have examined the origins of race-based medicine, the harm race-based medicine inflicts on minority bodies through race-based experimentation, and the false solutions a race-based drug ensues within minority communities. Such topics analyze the minority patient in a physical proxy. However, the mind and body are important entities, we cannot forget about the spirit. Healing is not just a physical practice; it includes spiritual practice. Efficient medicine includes the holistic elements of the mind, body, and spirit. Therefore, the spiritual discipline of black theology can be used as a tool to mend the harms of race-based medicine. It can be an avenue of research to further particular concerns about justice in medical care. Such theology contributes to the discussion of race-based medicine indicating the need for the voice, participation, and interdependence of minorities. Black theology can be used as a tool of healing and empowerment for health equity and awareness by exploring black theology's response to race-based medicine, analyzing race in biblical literature, using biblical literature as a tool for minority patient empowerment, building on past and current black church health advocacy with personal leadership in health advocacy.

© The Author(s) 2019
K. A. Johnson, *Medical Stigmata*,
https://doi.org/10.1007/978-981-13-2992-0_5

Race and Scripture

Black Theology

The African American experience is the testimony of a group that unfortunately went through inhumane, social, political, spiritual, economic, and other systemic injustices through lived experiences rooted within American race relations. These realities reflect the lived experience of an oppressed and marginalized group. Thus, "black" or "blackness" is not just a symbol of oppression, but of empowerment and endurance through the influence of black theology and its use in the black church.

The black church was created in response to the fight against discrimination and ongoing dehumanization. African Americans used to share houses of worship with whites, but they were not treated as valued children of God. Blacks wanted a place where they could worship freely without being monitored or dehumanized. Worship for African Americans became a means of survival. It was a chance to come together, as a community, and restore strength and hope in a racially cruel society. This is what the late Dr. James H. Cone describes as a "survival theology" in the black community. For Dr. Cone, "theology cannot be separated from the community which it represents."[1] This truth has been evident ever since the establishment of slavery and it is the duty of African Americans to evaluate the implications of their experience and to be consistent in its commitment to defend its existence.

Black theology "analyzes the oppression of black people, affirms the personhood of black people, and advocates their social and political liberation."[2] It is an extraordinary task to survive in a situation where one's inevitable and unchanging physical appearance, "one's blackness," is the cause of disease in a racially aggressive society. Because of such racial realities, race-based medicine continues to sustain the labels of race in society and medicine. Black theology gives minorities a voice asserting skin color does not affirm one's inferiority or bondage. Furthermore, it asserts skin color is not a marker to illness. As Dr. Miguel A. De La Torre suggests,

"Liberation is not just a symbol, it should mean a radical break with the status quo designed to maintain oppressive structures."[3] Black theology as survival theology is a response to the labels of race and illness by liberating the minority community to participate and speak out against the stigma of racial disease.

Black theology is a tool that demonstrates multiple black perspectives and experiences. By contrast, race-based medicine encourages a truncated look at black experiences. To fully understand the black experience, one must be black. The black experience is fully understood and realized by black persons. This does not mean the black experience is totally homogenous. The black experience is diverse through its unique cultures, languages, and historical discourse. Rather, recognizing the complexity of pathology and epidemiology in a racial group, race-based medicine encapsulates the black illness narrative in general terms. Dr. Cone mentions WEB DuBois comment that the black soul is not learned, "it comes from the *totality* of black experience, the experience of carving out an existence in a society that says you do not belong" (emphasis Added).[4] Race-based medicine does not look at the totality of the African American pathological experience rather it irrationally uses drugs as a quick fix toward health equity.

In a social context, African Americans are still in an inescapable degradation. African Americans know their physical blackness was constructed never to be an appropriate form of human existence. The construction of African Americans being less human is the affirmation of whatever is considered degrading, because the idea of orthodoxy is "whiteness." Race-based medicine reasserts the negative ideologies and theologies of skin color. As Dr. Delores S. Williams mentions, "The Bible and white interpretations of biblical stories also fed into this debasement of blackness and black people."[5] Due to harmful social and biblical interpretations, blacks call themselves beautiful, because a racist society and churches made "blackness" ugly. Blacks glorify blackness because it is despised. The black experience is catching the spirit of blackness and loving it. It is the powerful tool of self-love and affirmation that sustained the value of black skin and black self-worth.

In a political context, Dr. De La Torre describes, "If the dominant culture continues to be the sole interpreter of moral reality, then its perspectives will continue to be the norm by which the rest of society is morally judged."[6] The framework of "law and order" is the stability of the status quo. This results in putting blacks in a political box by "staying in their place", and the "moral" and "political" obligation "whiteness" to be a social standard. The black experience is more than dealing with racism. It means blacks are empowered to make decisions about themselves and have the autonomy to fulfill their decisions and desires. Race-based medicine hinders autonomy by restricting racial groups' choices and identification.

Race was a means of identification, as a means to classify and separate one group from the next. As Dr. Cornell West states, "Identity has to do with protection, association and recognition. People identify themselves in certain ways in order to protect their bodies, their labor, their communities, and their way of life."[7] The fact that the black community, at one point, did not have a collective sense of self made it easier for those individuals that were anti-black to take advantage of them. The manipulation of the African American community's social protection was a result of lost recognition and association. One might assume race-based medicine promotes recognizing disadvantaged groups affected by health inequity. However, it does the complete opposite. Race-based medicine continues the racist language of labels and stereotypes exclusively associating medical conditions and diseases to a racial group. The development of black power (African American self-determination as agents of social and political change) challenged the ideologies of race-based medicine by empowering the black community to define its own place and value. The use of black power and black theology aided in developing a positive perception of being black.

The concept of black power brought self-esteem and self-respect to the African American community. Black power was an efficient means of participatory theology and bioethics in the black community. As Dr. Lisa S. Cahill suggests, "Theological bioethics as participatory must explicitly link religion and theology to practices and movements in civil society that can have a subversive or revolutionary impacts on liberalism, science, and the market."[8] Black power was influential because it enabled African Americans to take a self- assessment of their value. It was evident that race-based medicine does not value and label the African American, but if African Americans do not value themselves; than they truly do not have self-value. Black power teaches one that true value comes from oneself not others and black theology brought spiritual relevance to self-value. Both were powerful mechanisms that kept African Americans sane and gave hope for temporal and eternal justice.

Black theology defines empowerment and justice of African Americans in an environment that is rooted in and thrives on oppression. However, black theology is not solely based upon what whites did to blacks, but a symbol of justice for everyone who are oppressed. It is an extension of progressive action for anyone who are victims of the status quo. Black theology is participation theology that, "holds up as an explicit goal, the creation of connective practices among interlocutors in order that shared social practices may be transformed in light of religiously inspired … visions and values."[9]

Blacks replaced dehumanizing identifications with the belief that they were created by God with equal value. Black theology condemns race-based medicine because it separates racial groups as different beings through the construction of race. It does not matter what skin color one possesses; we are all human beings and come from the same God. Race should not determine the proxy of disease. Therefore, it is African Americans' human rights to be treated with dignity and respect by the virtue of their creation.

The historical accumulations of racism, xenophobia, segregation, slavery, and a perverted form of Christianity tainted diversity. Blacks lived through serious consequences, oppressive conditions, and unimaginably traumatic experiences, thus making black skin a relevant physical trait based on historical experience. African Americans comprehend their identity by connecting symbols of the past. The black experience, good and bad, shaped what blackness signifies. Race-based medicine reasserts racist ideologies in medical discourse. As a result, labels oppress minority communities, minorities' personhood is challenged, and the adequate alleviation of health inequity will not be addressed.

Identity

As discussed in Chapter 1, race is a social and historical construction that corrupted social ideologies in the United States. This was evident through numerous xenophobic actions. Xenophobia is an unreasonable fear, distrust, or hatred of strangers, foreigners, or anything perceived as foreign or different. This was the behavior of the United States and its European influence. European society did not adequately comprehend African and Caribbean societies and the defense mechanisms of fear and lack of understanding soon became realities. So, as a result, "white" society rendered identity as a comfort zone, and fashioned a social spectrum, in the new world to emphasize its own self-worth, and magnify difference.

The self-worth of "whiteness" evolved into a repulsive and conceited pride called white supremacy, which resulted in Jim Crow laws, and the unscientific and irrational declaration of Social Darwinism, which lead to the biological, medical, and social degrading of minorities. As Cornel West states, "Oftentimes they [blacks] were not welcome in white suburbs, and they weren't being recognized. Their talents and capacities were debased, devalued and degraded."[10] These elements and principles of thought brought about the social construct of race created by the fear of human difference.

Blackness is not a certainty inscribed by genetics, fundamental human difference, or biological traits, but an actuality through historical experience. Through racial discourse, racial denigration slowly developed. This persuasion quickly developed in the early years of the United States. White social development became the standard (the idea of normalcy) in American society, thus, making race Americanized socially and historically. Blackness became an historical signifier of suffering and social injustice.

For example, when we define an object, we explain or identify the nature or essential qualities of the object. As long as, the object is immutable or unchangeable, the definition is the same. For example, we know that a tree is a plant having a permanently woody main stem or trunk, ordinarily growing to a considerable height, and usually developing branches at some distance from the ground. On the other hand, if the tree's trunk, branches, and leaves change; do we still call it a tree?

If the object possesses differences, but the essential qualities are the same, how will one conclude on identity? This is the same question we might ask about race. We are all human. External qualities are different, but humanness and value are no less due to external differences.

Jeremiah 13:23 states, "Can Ethiopians change their skin or leopards their spots? Then also you can do good who are accustomed to do evil." In context, the prophet Jeremiah is proclaiming to Judah that they cannot change their transgressions. As a result, they will have dire consequences. The wording of this text demonstrates perceptions of one's appearance. In contemporary understanding, Ethiopian should not be associated with the African country and its citizens. The term Ethiopians or Cushites (in other translations) refers to the color of a group of people's skin. It means blackness, dark or black skinned, Negro, or burnt skin complexion.[11] Misinterpretation of this scripture was used as a scientific biblical reference to assert the fatalism of racial traits and manipulated human beings as different racial entities.[12] Regardless of what skin color one possesses, it does not exclude one from being a viable human bring.

The object as we know as the human person has changed through self-manipulation. As Theologian Karl Rahner states, "Self-manipulation means that today man is changing himself."[13] Due to enhanced medical technology, a person can alter or change external qualities. Some examples are a person born a male can change into a female and vice versa, a veteran who lost limbs in a war can receive prosthetic limbs, differently abled individuals with mental challenges, and individuals with different hues of skin color. All these examples define the human person. The differences do not diminish any individual's humanness.

Difference compliments the complexities of being human. Personhood is complex. Extrinsic qualities can never provide a concrete definition, because they are unique and will change with time. The internal sense of humanity is invariable regardless of time. Self-manipulation happens when one changes the essence of who they are to conform to ideologies, dogmas, theologies, and social constructs that reject the uniqueness of their humanity. Hence, race-based medicine does not compliment social progression. Rather, it sustains the harmful notions about race. The relativism of what America conceived as "race" is also evident in what we classify as the human person. The definitions of a human being and race in our present age are far more complex than we originally thought and expressed in language.

Humanity is empowered by actions and choices. This freedom of choice or free will was exploited through Adam and Eve's disobedience (cf. Genesis 3). Their disobedience led to their existence as objects separate or apart from God's original intentions. Before the fall of mankind, Adam and Eve were in genuine assurance of who they were, but after the fall their God given essence was diminished. In the human race's compromised essence, we began to insert self-manipulation in the form of race. We became self-righteous believing we were more valuable than our human counterparts. Such egotistical realities perverted and constructed race by using monogenism and polygenism in biblical scripture.

Misunderstandings of Scripture

Based out of the Genesis etiology accounts, monogenism and polygenism were two schools of thought. Monogenism is the theory that the human race has descended from a single ancestral type. Polygenism suggests the human race has descended from two or more ancestral types. Polygenism is the belief ancestors from Adam were white individuals and other minorities were called pre-Adamites meaning before Adam. In 1520, the idea of polygenism first came from Swiss physician Paracelsus who believed that Adam's ancestors inhabited a small region in the earth and minorities came from a completely different origin.[14] The notion was God's first creation (minorities) was not sufficient, but God's second creation Adam and Eve (whites) was the perfect representation of creation. As Dr. Naomi Zack mentions, "polygenic theory of distinct origins for different races was used to argue that Africans, Asians, and Indians were permanently inferior to whites. That is, both the monogenicists and polygenicists began with the premise of white superiority, but differed about its nature."[15] Numerous debates on human geography and human origins were a part of monogenicists and polygenicists dialogue.

In 1591, Italian philosopher Giordano Bruno did not agree that black individuals came from the same origin of Jews. In 1655, a French protestant named Isaac de La Peyrere suggested pre-Adamite races produced Africa, Asia, and the New World.[16] New York lawyer William Frederick Van Amringe was cautious of pre-Adamite ideas in his 1848 publication called *Investigation of the Theories of the Natural History of Man*, but believed in multiple human species of different creative origins.[17]

In the early nineteenth century, a major figure in the study of skulls was Dr. Samuel George Morton. Morton collected and studied over 600 skulls to discover "that a ranking of races could be established objectively by physical characteristics of the brain, particularly by its size."[18] Based on his studies, Morton published *Crania Americana* (1839) and *Crania Aegyptiaca* (1844). Consequently, both of Morton's studies influenced the idea of monogenism and racial ranking. As Dr. Kaila Adia Story asserts, "European as well as American scientists not only were 'scientifically' invested in the conviction of African inferiority, but also created an ideology outlay with this assumption, due to their capitalist and social interests."[19] The pre-Adamite ideology was used to prove human variation.

Physician John Mason Good believed that different groups adapt to geography and were products of human variations. He claimed, "The first fall of man… did not take place till one hundred and twenty-nine years after the creation of Adam."[20] Good's suggestion implies that the fall of man was due to the consequences of the pre-Adamites. Polygenicist David Hume and Naturalist Georges Buffon believed blacks were apart of inferior races, but could improve being in the proper environments.[21] Swiss naturalist Harvard Louis Agassiz's two papers in the 1850 *Christian Examiner* proposed there are distinct zoological zones or provinces in which the creator placed discrete species and in his *Naturphilosophie* he asserted that each race had its point of origin.[22] Agassiz did not believe in the Genesis account, but suggested races were made for specific places.

Other individuals that promoted human variation included Boston medical naturalist Samuel Kneeland, who produced an 84 page intro in his 1848 *The Natural History of the Human Species*.[23] Arabic scholar and lexicographer Edward William Lane believed the pre-Adamite race existed during and after Adam and the Adamites' race were divinely created and mated with pre-Adamites to produce diversity of racial types. Baptist layman and physician George Moore attributed race to climate in his 1866 book *The First Man and His Place in Creation* and physical anthropologist James Cowles Prichard proclaimed a civilization as a race-forming factor that stimulated variation by the process of domestication.[24] Clinical psychologist Robert Dunn held the same belief that the environment modified skin color, hair and character. Polygenism was a means to justify and explain racial etiology and racist treatment, but such claims are not consistent with the historical and literary milieu of scripture.

The 1988 *Nature* article written by University of California at Berkeley scientists Dr. Mark Stoneking, Rebecca Cann, and Allan Wilson revealed unprecedented insight into the etiology of humanity. Their research uncovered the maternal ancestor of existing humans.[25] This figure was named "Mitochondrial Eve" or "African Eve." According to the article, Africans are the most diverse and Asians the next across all functional regions, which suggests that "Africa is a likely source of the human mitochondrial gene pool."[26] In the process of research, the Mitochondrial DNAs from 147 people were drawn from five geographic populations had been analyzed by restriction mapping. All the mitochondrial DNA came from one woman who is postulated to have lived about 200,000 years ago, in Africa. All populations were examined to have multiple origins, except African populations, implying that each area was colonized repeatedly.[27]

Such a discovery brings serious reservations about Paracelsus' racial pre-Adamite claims. To be fair, we have the benefit of science and technology that was not even imagined in the early sixteenth century. However, what this late twentieth century discovery challenged was the perceived "white washing" of biblical figures which has been ingrained in European and American biblical narrative for centuries, excluding positive biblical perceptions of African representation. The book of origins known as Genesis illustrated key racial passages that influenced racial discourse in American society.

Genesis 4:1–15 illustrates the first children in canonized scripture Cain and Abel. It appears that the first sexual act occurs outside of the garden, but this is not entirely clear. The name Cain (*qayin*) meaning "I have produced" (*qaniti*). Cain, the first older brother in the scriptures, is initially a tiller of the ground, like his father (Adam), continuing the troubled relationship between man (*'adam*) and the ground (*'adamah*). This difficulty is based from his father's disobedience in the Garden of Eden (cf. Genesis 3:14–19). Abel, the younger son, like King David in his youth was the keeper of the ship, which had less prestige than farming.

Genesis 4:3–7 continues with Yahweh's interaction with Cain and Abel's offering. The only difference between the values of the two sacrifices is that Abel offers the "firstlings," in contrast to Cain who offers the fruit (but not the first fruit). The text implies that Abel gave the freshest offering, and Cain gave God the leftovers.[28] Cain's interaction with Abel resulted in Abel's death. When Yahweh asked Cain, Where is your brother Abel? Cain's profound response was, "Am I my brother's keeper?" This is the first question that a human being had ever asked God in the biblical canon. Cain's answer has become a question of arrogance, selfishness, and disownment. This question comes from the same lips that shared the same milk from their mother Eve's breast, and now the same thing that sustained them, the milk from the same source, which bounded them together in their brotherhood, has now turned sour. Sour milk tainted by a selfish and jealous mentality. The pain caused by Cain's selfishness and jealousy caused him to kill his brother.

In an American context, the realities of fear (xenophobia) are the elements that divide humanity. It causes us to think that one is racially better or worse off than our fellow human equals. God created us and shaped us in his image (*imago dei*), and breathed into us the spirit of life. As humans, we tainted our God given skin colors, and react just like Cain. Like spoiled milk, our human harmony became sour and human diversity devalued. As a result, we now find ourselves asking the question "Am I my brother's keeper?" Am I responsible for my brother or sister regardless of what they look like, and what social context they are situated in? Consequently, members in our society answer with mythic attitudes of racial pride.

Further on, in verses 10 through 15, God and Cain's had a discussion,

And the Lord said, 'What have you done? Listen; your *brother's blood is crying out to me* from the ground! And now you are *cursed from the ground*, which has opened its mouth to receive your brother's blood from your hand. When you till the ground, it will no longer yield to you its strength; you will be a fugitive and a wanderer on the earth.' Cain said to the Lord, 'My punishment is greater than I can bear! Today you have driven me away from the soil, and I shall be hidden from your face; I shall be a fugitive and a wanderer on the earth, and anyone who meets me may kill me.' Then the Lord said to him, 'Not so! Whoever kills Cain will suffer a sevenfold vengeance.' And the Lord put a *mark on Cain*, so that no one who came upon him would kill him. (emphasis added)

The polygenistic hermeneutics of this text asserted that Cain was cursed with the mark of black skin. As Dr. Charles B. Copher suggests, "Cain as an ancestor of black peoples is the pre-Adamite view."[29]

Ancient rabbis developed two interpretations about Cain's blackness. The first suggests that Cain became black because of the smoke from his sacrifice or Cain's face became black because of hail.[30] This interpretation is extremely disjointed. The text illustrates Cain's response was fearful, because he believed that his punishment was unbearable, and his life would be in danger. In response, God gave Cain a mark of protection to prevent Cain from enduring physical harm or threat. The text does not inherently illustrate anything about Cain's mark being a change in his skin color. Since the twelfth century, interpretations of Cain's change in skin color have been associated with European hermeneutics.[31]

Like his father Adam, Cain's curse was from the earth or ground. Cain's mark was a bestowal of grace dealing with his punishment not the punishment itself. Furthermore, the text demonstrates that God found out about Abel's murder not by Cain confessing, but through a disembodied cry for justice.

God's profound statement to Cain echoes, "if the body is not present, the body's blood cries out for one's defense." Abel's blood stains on the ground were a representation of his identity and visual evidence of Cain's immoral act. This mirrors the countless bloodshed of black bodies by the institution of slavery, Jim Crowism, lynchings, medical experimentations, race riots, and police brutality are not forgotten. Throughout the centuries, black bodies through blood, sweat, and tears have been crying out for justice. Black ancestors are gone, but their blood still speaks through liberating theology, advocacy, and protest.

Genesis 9:18–27 illustrates the experience of Noah's nakedness and the curse of Canaan. I suggest three important elements in this text. First, Noah's nakedness, second, covering or hiding Noah's nakedness, and third turning away or ignoring Noah's nakedness. Noah's nakedness is interchangeable with sin (transgression). There is also a sexual element in this text, but I will digress from this topic since my focus is race. The Ark was a symbol of the new world, and a fresh start, but Noah and Ham tainted such new beginnings.

Noah abused his power and free will by excessive drinking. Instead, of turning away immediately and covering Noah, Ham saw Noah in a state he was not supposed to see him in, which violated two norms highly stressed in the Tanakh and Rabbinic Judaism, bodily modesty and the norm to honor and respect one's parents (cf. Exodus 28; 20:12, Leviticus 19). Out of guilt, Ham called Shem and Japheth, who walked backwards to cover Noah. Shem and Japheth walking backwards is a suggested representation of stagnating human-kind's progress.

Genesis 9:24–27 records the curse of Canaan, which has been notoriously and inappropriately used as a demeaning interpretation of race. The transgression of American Church history was the misappropriation of this text. As the late Rev. Dr. Katie G. Cannon observes, "Central to the whole hermeneutical approach was a rationalized biblical doctrine positing the innate and permanent inferiority of Blacks in the metonymical curse of Ham."[32] The curse of Ham or Canaan was used as biblical justification to enslave black folks who were viewed as the "Sons of Ham." Through polygenistic interpretation, Ham and Cain's descendants were revealed by their black skin as a physical representation of both curses.

Similar to Noah being the father of nations in the new ancient world, the fathers of the proposed new world called America perverted their free will and abused their power. American forefathers enforced excessive inhumane and unethical treatment of those from Africana descent. As Dr. Sylvester A. Johnson notes, "The Hamitic was unyieldingly wed to the institution of slavery because American slavery was preeminently racial. Its victims were exclusively the folk whose existence was already popularly explained in terms of Hamitic descent."[33] As a result, millions of black folks could not reach their full human potential. American nakedness (transgression) permeated through generations of injustice.

Instead of exposing one's history of racial relations, America brought its "Shem and Japheth" type of response that "God would 'enlarge' Japheth, putatively by ensuring that whites would succeed 'Shemites' and become bearers of religious truth and Ham was to have served them both."[34] America's actions of denial and the status quo walking backwards, hindering progress, covering up its transgressions through filtered media and educational structures that hide and skew information, knowledge, and history. Then blame the state of black individuals on themselves not acknowledging historical domestic neglect on black societies. Simultaneously, America's face turns away, because it refuses to see its own neglect of black lives. Such realities make the survival of blacks a reality using black theology.

Contrary to polygenetic views, black theological interpretation of Hebrew scripture illustrated endearing situations about figures of African descent. For example, Numbers 12:1–15 is an account of Moses and his Ethiopian or Cushite wife. Aaron and Miriam had reservations about Moses marrying a dark-skinned woman. As a result, God punished Miriam with leprosy as white as snow (v. 10). This text has dual meanings. First, whiteness suggested as a negative symbol or a curse. Second, blackness represented a gain of class and status.

The text spurs interest in the explicit phrase "leprous, as white as snow." For example, Isaiah 1:18 states, "Come now, let us argue it out, says the Lord: though your sins are like scarlet, they shall be like snow; though they are red like crimson, they shall become like wool." As Dr. Randall C. Bailey asserts,

The interpretation rests upon the understanding that in the Hebrew canon to be white as snow is a curse. Being made white as snow in Isaiah is often mistranslated. For Bailey, "Such is seen in the oft-mistranslated Isaiah 1:18. In this verse, part of a judgment speech, the charge begins with the word 'm, 'if.' Thus, the prophet proclaims, 'Come to judgment, if your sins are as scarlet [= negative], then they will be made white as snow [= the punishment]. Since all other instances of 'm found in this unit are read as 'if,' there appears to be no reason, other than the desire to keep the phrase 'white as snow' as a blessing, to translate it here as 'contrary to fact/though,' as do most exegetes. The punishment for complaining about Cushites as a means of status makes her the exact opposite of the Cushite, white as snow.[35]

God's response illustrated Miriam's important social standing of that time. Dr. Renita J. Weems asserts, "Her reputation as a poet and songstress (Exodus 13:21), combined with her anointing as a charismatic leader (Micah 6:4), must have made Miriam a figure to be reckoned with by the Hebrews, especially among women."[36] Also, Jeremiah's account illustrated a positive narrative of a Cushite named Ebedmelech who rescued the prophet Jeremiah (cf. Jeremiah 38:7–13).

The New Testament mentions positive stories of ancient black individuals, which serves as biblical representations of empowerment. For example, Simone of Cyrene helped Jesus carry his cross (cf. Mark 15:21). Cyrene was an ancient city in Libya, Africa. Simon is suggested to be the model disciple because he "literally took up the cross" to assist Jesus, which deemed his action "justifiable under the rules of Greco-Roman rhetoric."[37] Even John of Patmos described Jesus Christ with white hair like lamb's wool (nappy hair) and feet like polished brass (cf. Revelation 1:14–15). Jesus was not a white individual, but came from African and Asian ancestry.[38] Scriptures like these were used by the black preacher to discourage anti-black usage of scripture. The Black theology in scripture is a powerful tool for minority patient empowerment.

Biblical and Medical Narrative: Empowerment and Justice

As discussed in the three previous chapters, race-based medicine excludes and limits the holistic possibilities of care for minority patients. Scripture can be used as an effective aid for empowerment using illness narratives in the gospels. New Testament illness narratives are the experiences of Jesus Christ interacting with individuals or groups that are suffering from illness, disease, and deformity. I will use the illness narratives of the leper in Galilee (cf. Mark 1:40–45), the man with a withered hand in a synagogue at Capernaum (cf. Mark 3:1–7), and the woman with the issue of blood at Capernaum (cf. Mark 5:24–34)[39] as a means of minority patient empowerment.

Leper in Galilee

Mark 1:40–45 illustrates the first time Jesus heals from the ancient disease of Leprosy. Other accounts of leprosy were in the gospel of Luke (cf. Luke 5:12–14; 17:11–19). The text does not specifically mention where Jesus was. Jesus enters this unknown village and comes across a leper who approaches him. He begs to be cured from his leprosy.[40] Leprosy is a contagious disease that affects the skin, mucous membranes, and nerves, causing discoloration and lumps on the skin and, in severe cases, disfigurement and deformities. According to the *Oxford Dictionary of English*, leprosy is now mainly confined to tropical Africa and Asia. In biblical times, there was no treatment for leprosy. Today, leprosy can be cured with different form of antibiotics.

In a begging posture, the leper knelt and said, "If you choose, you can make me clean." This was significant because the leper approached Jesus. Lepers lived a life being perceived to have no dignity and value. They did not receive any sympathy from the community and society they existed in. For years, they saw individuals come and go that could not help them in their leprous condition. They were often feared to cause a major epidemic, which would threaten the survival of ancient society. That is why most lepers kept their distance because Jewish law required them to stay away from non-leprous individuals to prevent the spread of disease and to prevent the defiling of sacred buildings like the Tabernacle and religious gatherings (cf. Leviticus 13:46; Numbers 5:2–3).

Yet, this individual broke all social and religious norms to be cured from his disease. Jesus, being a Jewish Rabbi, also broke Jewish law by interacting with him. Jesus had empathy on him and healed the man. Jesus was not concerned with the social and religious etiquette. He acknowledged the humanity of the individual. In humility, Jesus urged the leper not to report his holistic experience. Of course, the leper who had been cured from his disease told everyone he could. He received his autonomy, value, and integrity with one experience of ethical care. He was empowered to thrive in a society that ostracized him for so long because of the peculiarity of his skin.

Similar to the leper's experience, the minority patient had been devalued because of his or her skin. As described in Chapters 1 and 2, black skin was viewed as a medical and social threat to American society. It was an epidemic associated with sickle cell anemia and other diseases. Blacks were forced to keep their distance from whites because of what they looked like. I suggest black skin was (and still is) the stigmata of medicine.

Stigmata is the term used for the marks of Jesus Christ's crucifixion, which were the marks on Christ's head (crown of thorns), hands and feet (nails), and side (spear). The Apostle Paul mentions that he bears the marks of Christ (cf. Galatians 6:17). Stigmata refers to the suffering of Jesus Christ's crucifixion and victory of his resurrection. In contrast, black skin as "medical stigmata" symbolizes the suffering of black people in unethical clinical treatment and the victory of overcoming such monstrosities through advocacy.

It is unfortunate that health disparities and mediocre medical treatment continue to affect African Americans. As Dr. Emilie M. Townes suggests, "The US medical system suffers from interstructered paternalism and racism. One of the foundational aspects of this problem is the way many doctors receive their training and the lack of rigorous and ethically responsible clinical trials that include racial-ethnic men and women and white women."[41] As I addressed in Chapter 3, clinical solutions can start with physician training in cultural competency, empathy and awareness. However, this was not a reality for African Americans throughout most of the twentieth century. African Americans had to develop their own means of health and wellness. Blacks built adequate medical care through the legacy of the Black Panther Party.

The Black Panther Party (BPP) was notorious for its brash response to a racist society. The organization was widely known for its political activism, but the BPP was also instrumental in health advocacy and outreach. BPP's advocacy was reflected through the People's Free Medical Clinics (PFMCs). The clinic's goal was to have "completely free health care for all black and oppressed people."[42] PFMCs operated through community based medical clinics and a health network of professionals.

For most of the twentieth century, it was very difficult for blacks to get medical care because public hospitals were often overcrowded and lacked adequate staff and private hospitals were too expensive. The PFMCs provided the means for African Americans to get efficient care in their local communities. Individuals with serious medical needs or surgery were suggested to go to doctors and medical facilities that would be able to assist. The leper's story demonstrated Jesus Christ's empathy and solidarity toward the leper while completely disregarding societal norms and rules. PFMCs philosophy was "Christ like" bringing humanism within medical care. It represented empathic care inclusive of socioeconomic status and acceptance. PFMCs asserted health care as a human right and not a commodity.

The Party's PFMCs rebuilt the patient-physician relationship in the black community. Historical perceptions of American medicine reflected the symbol of the white coat as a symbol of suffering and even death in communities of color. However, the important element of trust for blacks in the medical clinic was restored through PFMCs. As Sociologist Dr. Alondra Nelson states,

> The white coat of medical science could have a different connotation in black communities. Because the Party worked with populations that historically had not had regular contact with medical professionals, the white coat, worn by *trusted experts*, could be a welcome sign of long sought access to quality healthcare as well as an emblem of the potential *excesses of medical power.* (emphasis added)[43]

When the black community started to trust their medical professionals, they began to invest in a cause that genuinely invested in them. African Americans finally had the opportunity to go to someone who looked like them and understood black life. PFMCs gave blacks the authority to own their medical care and empowered them to take charge of their health.

All BPP clinics had examination tables, offered primary, preventive, and dental care, collaborated with medical professionals, conducted protocol for the spread of diseases, relied on donations for supplies and labor, and ran an ambulance EMT unit, which was provided by businesses, churches, and BPP's supporting organizations.[44] The clinics had grocery giveaways for individuals that did not have the means to buy food. PFMCs promoted health literacy and education. It also advocated for self-help care or self-care which trained women to do gynecological self-examinations and self-help testing for individuals with sickle cell anemia.[45]

Like the leper's enthusiastic response of his physical renewal, African Americans could not lay stagnant on their medical progress. PFMCs grew to a national level and influenced medical discourse. Blacks had to simultaneously continue to take charge of their health and be empowered to be active agents of change in American healthcare. PFMCs dwindled away in the 1970s, but its influence remains strong today through the health advocacy of the NAACP, Association of Black Cardiologists, the Congressional Black Caucus, the National Baptist Convention USA Inc.'s Health Outreach Prevention Education (HOPE) among many other organizations.

The Man with a Withered Hand

Mark 3:1–7 records Jesus Christ's interaction with a man that had issue with his hand. The Markan account described the condition of the man's hand as withered. It is obvious that we cannot precisely diagnose what ailment this man had. However, the man's condition can be suggested to be similar to Hand Atrophy (deterioration of muscles), severe Carpal Tunnel Syndrome (nerve issues that result in stiffness in hand and fingers), or a symptom of Cerebral Palsy (clamping of the hand).

The text described Jesus entered in a synagogue. His immediate attention was to a man with a withered hand. This event was on a sacred day, the Sabbath. Jewish law did not allow Jesus to perform any type of work. The Pharisees watched to see what Jesus' reaction was going to be. He either would not cure the man to conform to Jewish law or cure the man against Jewish law. The Pharisees took the Jewish Sabbath law very seriously and would reprimand Jesus if he broke the law. Jesus told the man who had the withered hand, "Come forward." While the Pharisees watched, Jesus told them, "Is it lawful to do good or to do harm on the Sabbath, to save life or to kill?"

The Pharisees, however, had no reply to Jesus' question. Jesus was angry about the Pharisees' unempathetic response and said to the man, "Stretch out your hand." The man stretched out his hand and was restored. The Pharisees wanted to punish Jesus for breaking the Sabbath law. Jesus retreated to the Sea of Galilee with his disciples where he was followed by spectators that witnessed the man's healing. This text demonstrates three critical evaluations. First, the synagogue, a place that should practice the concept of renewal did not. Second, practitioners of presence and compassion (the Pharisees) did not show it. Third, Jesus did not follow religious correctness to heal a man with a physical issue.

A synagogue is a place of healing, renewal, growth, learning, and understanding. Contrary to what we might initially think, a hospital should share the same attributes. It should be a place of holistic healing where anyone can practice their religious beliefs and spirituality without being compromised. Unfortunately, the man did not experience healing. The synagogue authorities (Pharisees) were so caught up in religious correctness that they failed to see the synagogue as a place of healing and renewal. No law or idea should be able to hinder a person's renewal and diminish their human value. This man's experience has been embodied through the black community through hospital care.

Chapter 2 mentioned the struggle of African Americans being able to get hospital care. Slave houses were the locations used to facilitate blacks' medical needs. Similar to the man with the withered hand, blacks were denied access for physical restoration or treated differently because of their racial status. As Dr. Aana M. Vigen states, "Doctors may not always see the actual person in front of them, but instead see only a generic representative of a larger group."[46] Blacks had to deal with racism and Jim Crow laws that prevented them to get healing in an institution that was created for such a purpose. As a result, there were not adequate hospitals to treat the black community, but that changed with exceptional insight of Dr. Daniel Hale Williams.

In 1891, Dr. Williams founded the Chicago's Provident Hospital and Nurse Training School.[47] It was the first black controlled hospital. Black hospitals treated African Americans with respect and dignity. In other hospitals, race mattered more than class in the quality of care a patient received. The fear of medical experimentation, death, discrimination, and mistrust embolden blacks to want their own hospitals. African Americans experienced value and compassion interacting with doctors who understood black life in American society. Williams made a national declaration for black owned hospitals. Williams' decree did not only involve hospitals to care for the sick, but also a means for medical education for black doctors and nurses who had very few options to practice medicine.

Kansas City General Hospital No. 2, also known as KC Colored Hospital, was the first major hospital for black patients with white staff. Dr. Thomas C. Unthank founded two small private hospitals Douglass Hospital in Kansas City, Kansas in 1898 and Lange Hospital in Kansas City, Missouri, in 1903.[48] In 1914, Kansas City General was the first hospital to be managed by an African American when Dr. William J. Thompson became the Superintendent and Mary K. Hampton-Brown named Superintendent of nurses. Ten years later all departments had black leadership. Other black controlled hospitals included Tuskegee Institute and Nurse training school in Alabama stabled in 1892; Fredrick Douglass Memorial Hospital and Training School in Philadelphia, established in 1895; and Home Infirmary Clarksville, Tennessee, established in 1906.[49] In 1912, 63 black controlled hospitals existed, and by 1919 almost, doubled to 118.[50]

Black hospitals thrived on the same mentality of the man with the withered hand. If a person has a chance to realize hope and achieve restoration, one's humanity and capacity for help should surpasses any law, ideology and theology. This was the testament of black hospitals. Throughout the twentieth century, black hospitals have closed due to financial strains and buyouts. There are only two black hospitals left. The Chicago Provident Hospital known as Provident Hospital of Cook County was taken over by the Cook County Bureau of Health Services and Howard University Hospital in Washington, DC.[51]

The Woman with the Issue of Blood

Mark 5:24–34 starts in a chaotic frenzy. A large crowd followed Jesus and surrounded him almost to the limit of asphyxiation. Amid the crowd, there was a woman who had been suffering from hemorrhages for twelve years. She tried many physicians and suffered painful experiences with her condition. She expunged all her financial resources, but gotten worse instead of getting better. However, this woman had hope because Jesus was in the area. When she saw him, she went through every tight space and crevice. Finally, she was close to him. She came up behind him in the compacted crowd and touched his cloak. In a determined response she said, "If I but touch his clothes, I will be made well."

The text immediately revealed that her hemorrhaging stopped, and she felt in her body that she was healed of her disease. Jesus noticed someone touched him. He turned about in the crowd and said, "Who touched my clothes?" His disciples responded, "You see the crowd pressing in on you; how can you say, 'Who touched me?'" Jesus looked around to see who touched him. The woman, who was now cured of her hemorrhaging approach Jesus reluctantly, fell and confessed she touched him. Jesus told her, "Daughter, your faith has made you well; go in peace, and be healed of your disease." This account was an example of Jesus, the feminist, challenging the customs and laws regarding women. As Dr. Jacquelyn Grant states, "Jesus elevated many who were at the bottom of the social hierarchy to a new level of equality. This trend is especially evident in his relationship with women."[52] Jesus' ministry had deep roots including women.

The woman with her hemorrhage issue shared experiences like enslaved women with vesico-vaginal fistula (VVF). They both had medical conditions that could not be cured, suffered years with the same condition before being cured, and experienced being outcasts in a male dominated society. The bleeding woman was viewed unclean because of the Jewish law of *niddah*. This law is referred to uterine bleeding not due to injury or trauma and its usual causes are through menstruation, bleeding during pregnancy or birth (*yoledet*), ovulation, and irregular flow of blood (*zavah*). This law prohibited any contact until the bleeding stops. After seven days with no bleeding, she will be immersed in a kosher ritual bath (*mikveh*). After the woman fulfilled the requirements of *niddah* law, all interactions are permitted until she anticipates bleeding to reoccur (cf. Leviticus 15:19–30; 18:19; 20:18).

The Markan text illustrates the bleeding woman had suffered with her condition for twelve years, which means she probably did not have any physical contact and interaction with anyone during that period of time. Her financial status was dire because she had no money and was disadvantaged earning money due to her sex. In addition, she was untouchable being viewed as unclean. Similar tones of distress come from enslaved black women. They were viewed unfit and unclean not because of a medical condition like VVF, but by the perceived inferiority of the color of their skin. Both women challenged by the societal limitations imposed on them.

The bleeding woman endured her medical condition under many physicians. Enslaved women endured numerous conditions under physicians who physically, mentally, and emotionally took advantage of them. For example, the unethical practices of Dr. J. Marion Sims discussed in Chapter 2. The bleeding woman's twelve year medical tribulation is horrific, but it fails in comparison with centuries of medical and civil abuses of enslaved women.

Yet, the bleeding woman and enslaved women received their healing through tenacious devotion to social change. The bleeding woman did not surrender because the crowd was compacted or tight around Jesus. Regardless of the difficulty, she found a way to position herself for healing. The bleeding woman had to overcome many obstacles in her twelve years of having hemorrhages, which shows her endurance and resolve. When the opportunity came for personal change and restoration, she took it by any means necessary.

This is an example of feminist theology. Dr. Grant mentions, "Because oppression tends to dehumanize its victims, women must reconceptualize ideas and images about themselves."[53] The woman in the text was tired of her physical condition and society's perception. She reframed her situation shifting from victim to victor. The woman transformed her social standing into an honorable woman of faith acknowledged by the great rabbi himself, Jesus Christ. The woman's reconceptualization was the same essence enslaved women used to influence American medicine through the importance of midwifery.

Midwifery is the procedure when a trained person assists women in childbirth. The practice of midwifery increased black women's social standing and mobility in slave communities. Midwives were able to travel around plantations on horseback, assist with the birth of slaveholders' children, and carry news without penalty.[54] Also, black midwives were able to visit family and friends. After slavery, midwives continued to play an important role in women's and public health. They promoted maternal-child prevention by giving encouragement for women to receive prenatal and postnatal care, notified nurses when a woman gave birth, and were liaisons between poor black women and white health professionals.[55]

Black midwives continued to empower their communities by controlling the spread of diseases and encouraging their communities to get tested for current disease threats. For example, African American midwives helped control the spread of venereal disease and syphilis by urging pregnant women and local communities to get blood tests.[56] The influence of midwifery in the black community promoted health education, literacy, prevention, and organization. The model birthing room was an unprecedented contribution of black midwives. In the early 1930s, the Mississippi State Board of Health required midwives to educate their communities about the modern standard for childbirth requirements.[57] The midwives modern birthing room demonstrations educated future parents, communities, and health organizations on proper protocol and sterilization of a birthing room.

African American midwives are the quintessential example of empowerment and health advocacy. Their knowledge and unique position in the black community pushed them to be voices of change. Black women used the profession of midwifery for social justice. They transformed their own clinical experience. Black women were the individuals being abused and mistreated in the clinical setting. As midwives, they help changed the status of black women from being recipients of maleficence and oppression to infusing a standard of care, empathy, and efficiency in gynecological and maternal care. Mark's account of the bleeding woman and black women in American medical history had to fight through encapsulating experiences being defined by sexist and racist societies. However, they overcame by achieved health advocacy and healing.

Black Church and Health Advocacy

Since its inception, the black church has been a spiritual, social, and political resource for the African American community. It has evolved into a resource of health advocacy in minority communities. The black church has progressively gotten better incorporating health education, literacy, and health partnerships within its congregations. However, there is still more work for the black church to do. This section reflects past and recent black church health advocacy movements and personal endeavors of health advocacy as a black clergy.

Early Movements in Black Church Health Advocacy

Historian and Sociologist Dr. WEB Du Bois established the first self-assessment of African American health in his 1906 publication *The Health and Physique of the Negro American*. It was part eleven out of an eighteen volume project dealing with multiple areas of black life including religion, economics, class and education.[58] The 136 page document was Du Bois' apologetic defense against social darwinism, polygenism, and eugenics' theories about race. He wanted to stress that race was not a fatalistic definition of disease. Health of human beings was the consequence of social, political, and environmental variables.

In Du Bois' landmark tuberculosis study, he retrieved vital statistics from the US Army recruiting examination records, life insurance companies, the US Bureau of the Census, and data of white working class groups in the United States and Europe, which concluded that, "Tuberculosis was not a racial disease, but a social disease linked to poverty, housing conditions, and working conditions."[59] Du Bois' research led the way for future black health initiatives and studies in secular and religious setting. Nine years later, the National Negro Health Week Movement began with the black church being its key resource.

From 1915 to 1951, the National Negro Health Week/Movement (NNHW/NNHM) encouraged blacks to advocate and address minority populations' health issues with the aptitude of health education and advocacy. The movement was founded by educator and founder of Tuskegee University Booker T. Washington. Initially, Washington's initiative was called "Health Improvement Week" an annual week of health awareness in early April, but the National Negro Business League (founded by Washington) with the financial sponsorship of industrialist Andrew Carnegie gave Washington the necessary financial support to make it a national initiative.[60]

The United States Public Health Service (USPHS) promoted NNHW into a national black health initiative. In 1921, the USPHS started to publish the National Negro Health Week Bulletin and had the US Surgeon General Dr. Hugh Smith Cumming convene at the first NNHW annual conference in Washington, DC.[61] In 1932, the National Negro Health Week became the National Negro Health Movement (NNHM) by the establishment of the Office of Negro Health Work through the USPHS.[62] The NNHM was supported by local health departments, civic groups, schools, media, and businesses. However, the grass roots advocacy of NNHW was the black church.

Sunday was the most important day for NNHW. The black church is an important institution in the black community because of its influence on change and transformation. On "Mobilization Sunday," black preachers exhorted health education sermons at worship services and church meetings.[63] NNHW organizers urged the usage of good speakers and music to keep the black community engaged and knowledgeable on health issues. Also, Sunday was "Reports and Follow-up Day" when the black community gathered at houses of worship for large civic meetings.

NNHW's schedule as follows: Monday "Home Hygiene Day," Tuesday "Community Sanitation Day," Wednesday "Special Campaign Day" which focused on specific local health needs, Thursday "Adult Health Day," Friday "School Health Day," and Saturday "General Cleanup Day," which was "the large scale cleanup activities and inspection of community health campaign results."[64] Sunday culminated in activates and goals of the week. The black church was the major conduit between the NNHW and the black community. The NNHW wanted to promote the church as its key partner. In 1933, a *NNHW News* editorial declared, "The church can render a most helpful service in the Health Week Anniversary by making occasional announcements and by starting the health week proper with a good message to the church assemblies all day."[65] An example of the NNHM communal success was Detroit, Michigan's Daniel Hale Williams Health Guild.

The Daniel Hale Williams Health Guild had 200 active participants who were all black women. The members of the Health Guild used the popularity of NNHM to get support from clergy, teachers, Detroit's Department of Health and physicians. One of the Health Guild's major projects was, "an eight week health clinic held in black churches that immunized over 5000 children against diphtheria."[66] Also, in Richmond, Virginia, physicians gave health education lectures at 53 black churches reaching over 10,000 people and black churches provided adult and children clinics in their houses of worship.[67] After nineteen years under the USPHS, the move toward integration led to the dismantling of the Office of Negro Health Work and the National Negro Health Movement. Du Bois and Washington's influence set the standard of black health advocacy and how the black church can be an integral resource in the process of health equity. Black church health advocacy continued throughout the twentieth century.

In the civil rights era (1954–1968), African Americans continued to fight against the many systemic injustices they endured daily. Healthcare was still in the vision of the black community with The Rev. Dr. Martin Luther King as the leader of the movement. On March 25, 1966, Dr. King proclaimed, "Of all the forms of inequality, injustice in health care is the most shocking and inhumane."[68] This quote was taken from his famous speech at the Convention of the Medical Committee for Human Rights held in Chicago. Black preachers have always been at the forefront for health advocacy in the black community. Another example is The Reverend Jesse Jackson.

Recent Black Church Health Advocacy

Rev. Jesse Jackson's black church health advocacy was centered on the prevention of HIV/AIDS. Rev. Jackson used slogans, health education materials, and ideas for policy reform.[69] The push for HIV/AIDS awareness was successful incorporating slogans and health education in sermons and youth programs. Another HIV black church partnership was with the Churches United to Stop HIV (CUSH) established in 1999. CUSH was based out of Broward County, Florida. CUSH's objective was, "to include training faith-based leaders and congregations to develop HIV educational programs, outreach and referral services, and support programs for infected individuals and others affected by the epidemic. To meet these objectives, CUSH staff created a training manual, brochures and palm cards."[70]

CUSH was not a health initiative exclusively led by the black church. Black churches were included with churches from all socioeconomic backgrounds. CUSH has provided HIV prevention to over 32,000 people, trained for over 2850 faith leaders, and provided risk assessments for over 1000 people, counseling and testing for over 825 participants and technical assistance for 48 churches.[71] African American Immunologist Pernessa C. Seele developed an organization called the "Balm in Gilead" to assist black churches developing programs to efficiently educate congregations on AIDS.[72]

In regard to drugs, the National Conference on the Black Family/Community and Crack Cocaine partnered with Rev. Jackson to alleviate the use of drugs. Rev. Jackson's famous slogan, "Down with Dope! Up with Hope!"[73] was a catch phrase for the youth to take a moral responsibility against the dangers of drugs. The National Conference on the Black Family/Community and Crack Cocaine involved 1200 churches from different denominations and health care professionals.[74] In 2000, the

Congress of Black Churches anti-drug and violence campaigns in 37 cities, with almost 2000 clergy members reaching out to 500,000 people and the Project Anti-Drug Abuse Movement (ADAM) consisted of 100 churches that provided health education on drug abuse.[75] HIV/AIDS and drug abuse are areas of national involvement for the black church. However, cardiovascular health is another national focus.

The Progressive National Baptist Convention (PNBC) has partnered with the National Cancer Institute (NCI). PNBC's program through the NCI is called "Body and Soul," which involves 1100 black churches in 22 states.[76] The Body and Soul is a nutrition program with the purpose of cardiovascular disease prevention. The National Baptist Convention USA, Inc. (NBCUSA, Inc.) developed the Health Outreach Prevention Education (HOPE), which I am an active clergy member.

H.O.P.E. is the National Baptist Convention U.S.A. Inc., Congress of Christian Education's Health Outreach and Prevention Education Initiative (H.O.P.E.). This program aims to bring health education, literacy, and programs to black communities as H.O.P.E. take actions that will dramatically improve health and positively impact total well-being. H.O.P.E. Initiative is a member of the national partnership for Action to End Health Disparities and the United States Department of Health & Human Services Office of Minority Health.

Black theology's response to race-based medicine is one of empowerment and justice. This results in the efficient holistic health of African Americans. Black individuals have the hope and encouragement of mental, physical, and spiritual well-being. Racist ideologies and theologies used biblical scripture as a weapon, but black liberation theology changed harmful interpretation to a means of self-pride. Such hermeneutical change was possible looking at the scripture from black experiences which allowed African Americans to create their own narrative in an unwelcoming society.

In American medicine, black hermeneutics gave African Americans the opportunity to associate biblical illness narratives to their own medical condition for hope to be restored and renewed. Furthermore, black theology and scripture inspired the black church to become self-reliant builders, organizers, administrators, educators, and advocates of black health. Such examples inspired a clergy like me to do what I can to fight against health disparities for those who still are not considered important. In comparison to race-based medicine, the black church and black theology are significant agents to mend the fragmented health of African Americans and are much more efficient in solving health issues in minority communities.

Notes

1. Cone, James. *A Black Theology of Liberation*. Philadelphia: Lippincott, 1970, 8.
2. Sanders, "European-American Ethos and Principlism," 78.
3. De La Torre, Miguel A. *Doing Christian Ethics from the Margins*. Maryknoll, NY: Orbis Books, 2004, 26.
4. Ibid., 25.
5. Williams, Delores S. *Sisters in the Wilderness: The Challenge of Womanist God-Talk*. Maryknoll, NY: Orbis Books, 1993, 91.
6. De La Torre, Miguel A. *Doing Christian Ethics from the Margins*. Maryknoll, NY: Orbis Books, 2004, 12.
7. West, Cornel. *Race Matters*. New York: Vintage Books, 1994, 501.
8. Cahill, Lisa Sowle. *Theological Bioethics*. Washington, DC: Georgetown University Press, 2005, 39.
9. Cahill, Lisa Sowle. *Theological Bioethics*. Washington, DC: Georgetown University Press, 2005, 38.
10. West, *Race Matters*, 501.
11. Sadler, Rodney S. "Can A Cushite Change His Skin? Cushites, 'Racial Othering' and the Hebrew Bible." *Interpretation* 60, no. 4 (2006), 390.
12. Washington, *Medical Apartheid*, 226.
13. Dych, William V. *Karl Rahner*. A&C Black, 2000, 134.
14. Graves, Joseph L. *The Emperor's New Clothes: Biological Theories of Race at the Millennium*. New Brunswick, NJ: Rutgers University Press, 2001, 25.
15. Zack, Naomi. *Philosophy of Science and Race*. New York: Routledge, 2002, 14.
16. Graves, *The Emperor's New Clothes*, 26.
17. Livingstone, David N. *Adam's Ancestors: Race, Religion, and the Politics of Human Origins*. Baltimore: Johns Hopkins University Press, 2008, 94.

18. Story, Kaila A. "Racing Sex-Sexing Race: The Invention of the Black Feminine Body." *Imagining the Black Female Body: Reconciling Image in Print and Visual Culture*, edited by Carol E. Henderson. New York: Palgrave Macmillan, 2010, 36.
19. Story, "Imagining the Black Female Body," 37.
20. Ibid.
21. Ibid., 30–31.
22. Ibid., 95.
23. Ibid., 97.
24. Livingstone, *Adam's Ancestors*, 117–119.
25. Oikkonen, Venla. "Mitochondrial Eve and the Affective Politics of Human Ancestry." *Signs* 40, no. 3 (2015), 748.
26. Stoneking, Mark, Rebecca L. Cann, and Allan C. Wilson. "Mitochondrial DNA and Human Evolution." *Nature* 325 (6099) (1987), 33.
27. Ibid., 32.
28. Gunn, D. M., and Danna Nolan Fewell. *Narrative in the Hebrew Bible*. New York: Oxford University Press, 1993, 15.
29. Copher, Charles B. "The Black Presence in the Old Testament." *Stony the Road We Trod: African American Biblical Interpretation*, edited by Cain Hope Felder. Minneapolis, MN: Fortress Press, 1991, 149.
30. Ibid., 148.
31. Ibid., 149.
32. Cannon, Katie G. "Slave Ideology and Biblical Interpretation." *The Recovery of Black Presence: An Interdisciplinary Exploration: Essays in Honor of Dr. Charles B. Copher*, edited by Charles B. Copher et al. Nashville: Abingdon Press, 1995, 121.
33. Johnson, Sylvester A. *The Myth of Ham in Nineteenth-Century American Christianity: Race, Heathens, and the People of God*. New York: Palgrave Macmillan, 2004, 70.
34. Ibid.
35. Bailey, Randall C. "Beyond Identification: The Use of Africans in Old Testament Poetry and Narratives." *Stony the Road We Trod: African American Biblical Interpretation*, edited by Cain Hope Felder. Minneapolis, MN: Fortress Press, 1991, 179–180.
36. Weems, Renita J. *Just a Sister Away: A Womanist Vision of Women's Relationships in the Bible*. San Diego, CA: LuraMedia, 1988, 72.

37. Sanders, Boykin. "In Search of a Face for Simon the Cyrene." *Stony the Road We Trod: African American Biblical Interpretation*, edited by Cain Hope Felder. Minneapolis: Fortress Press, 1991, 54.

38. Hopkins, Dwight N. *Down, Up, and Over: Slave Religion and Black Theology*. Minneapolis, MN: Fortress Press, 2000, 263.

39. The synoptic gospel of Mark is the earliest of the canonized gospels which is a personal preference of usage.

40. Biblical literature refers to this man's disease as leprosy. It is possible that this man had another disease. Since the pathology and diagnosis of diseases were not well known in ancient times, the word leprosy was used interchangeably to describe a condition not discovered or fully understood. To simplify, I will use the term leprosy for this man's condition.

41. Townes, Emilie Maureen. *Breaking the Fine Rain of Death: African American Health Issues and a Womanist Ethic of Care*. New York: Continuum, 1998, 45.

42. Nelson, *Body and Soul*, 4.

43. Nelson, *Body and Soul*, 84.

44. Nelson, *Body and Soul*, 84–90.

45. Ibid., 89–90.

46. Vigen, Aana Marie. *Women, Ethics, and Inequality in U.S. Healthcare: "To Count Among the Living."* New York: Palgrave Macmillan, 2006, 45.

47. Gamble, Vanessa Northington. *Making a Place for Ourselves: The Black Hospital Movement, 1920–1945*. New York: Oxford University Press, 1995, 11.

48. Gamble, *Making a Place for Ourselves*, 9.

49. Ibid., 11.

50. Ibid., 3.

51. Gamble, *Making a Place for Ourselves*, 194–195.

52. Grant, Jacquelyn. *White Women's Christ and Black Women's Jesus: Feminist Christology and Womanist Response*. Atlanta, GA: Scholars Press, 1989, 143.

53. Grant, *White Women's Christ and Black Women's Jesus*, 119.

54. Fett, *Working Cures*, 130.

55. Smith, Susan Lynn. *Sick and Tired of Being Sick and Tired: Black Women's Health Activism in America, 1890–1950*. Philadelphia: University of Pennsylvania Press, 1995, 140.

56. Ibid., 141.
57. Ibid., 144–145.
58. Nelson, *Body and Soul*, 45.
59. Ibid., 46–47.
60. Quinn, Sandra Crouse, and Stephen B. Thomas. "The National Negro Health Week, 1915 to 1951: A Descriptive Account." *Minority Health Today* 2, no. 3 (2001), 45.
61. Ibid., 46.
62. Nelson, *Body and Soul*, 30.
63. Quinn, "The National Negro Health," 46–47.
64. Quinn, "The National Negro Health," 46.
65. Ibid., 47.
66. Smith, *Sick and Tired*, 53.
67. Ibid., 63.
68. Peterson, Eric, and Clyde W. Yancy. "Eliminating Racial and Ethnic Disparities in Cardiac Care." *New England Journal of Medicine* 360, no. 12 (2009), 1172.
69. Pinn, Anthony B. *The Black Church in the Post-Civil Rights Era*. Orbis Books, 2002, 96.
70. Agate, Lisa L., D'Mrtri Cato-Watson, Jolene M. Mullins, Gloria S. Scott, Vanice Rolle, Donna Markland, and David L. Roach. "Churches United to Stop HIV (CUSH): A Faith-Based HIV Prevention Initiative." *Journal of the National Medical Association* 97, no. 7 (Suppl) (2005): 60S, 61S.
71. Ibid.
72. Pinn, *The Black Church*, 100.
73. Ibid., 96.
74. Ibid., 97.
75. Ibid.
76. DMin, William Booth. "Partnering with the Black Church: Recipe for Promoting Heart Health in the Stroke Belt." *ABNF Journal* 23, no. 2 (2012), 36.

6

Conclusion

Race-based medicine is an emerging field in pharmacology, a field which aims to create a specialty market based on racial groups. Within this field, the drug BiDil set precedents for this area of medicine, targeting African Americans as its first racial group. Immediately, the idea of race as a proxy for disease caused much debate within the medical and pharmaceutical communities. Furthermore, race-based medicine's "starter group" being African Americans caused ethical questions regarding the motive behind race-based medicine because of the treatment of blacks in American medical history. This conclusion will review and summarize the link between race-based medicine and American eugenics, race-based medicine's influence on the perception of the black body, the influence of BiDil's approval on the resurgence of race-based medicine, the black church's response to race-based medicine using black theology, and suggestions for future explorations of race-based medicine.

In Chapter 1, I discussed Jean Bapiste de Lamarck, an important figure in the foundation of eugenics. Lamarckism the foundation of the eugenics movement was also connected with polygenism and concepts of degeneration. Out of Lamarckism ideology, Charles Robert

© The Author(s) 2019
K. A. Johnson, *Medical Stigmata*,
https://doi.org/10.1007/978-981-13-2992-0_6

Darwin formulated concepts about evolution and natural selection in his popular work called *Origin of Species* which produced the field of Social Darwinism. Francis Galton developed the notion of eugenics into a field of science, which evolved into the area of positive and negative eugenics. Under the influences of Karl Pearson, Gregor Mendel, and Walter F. R. Weldon, Charles Davenport brought the practice of negative eugenics into American society and culture.

Davenport shaped the ideology and research paradigm of American eugenics. As a result, the Eugenics Record Office influenced the process of defining and classifying American society. Sociomedical racism became the norm, affecting individuals with Sickle Cell Anemia and Tay Sachs Disease. SCA and TSD were the diseases that spawned the idea of racial diseases. Specifically, SCA researchers created the assumptions that racial groups have different blood types. Such assumptions regarding race-based disease influenced American law and policy. Sterilization, birth control, marriage control, and immigration policies were rooted in the fear and control of race-based disease. The perception that racial groups are innately different formed biological and anatomical theories of difference, which developed into deceitful assertions about racial groups' physiology—especially the observations about African American bodies discussed in Chapter 2.

Chapter 2 overviewed the understanding of race and body representation in American history. African Americans were devalued through the misappropriation of their bodies. The dehumanizing denial of black personhood sustained a language and ideology of inferiority. Consequently, pseudo-biological claims compromised the autonomy of black citizens. Physician Samuel Cartwright advanced the understandings of black hardiness and black durability. Cartwright's influence expanded the research on race anomalies resulting in slavery, military, and prison race-based experimentation.

Slave experimentation consisted of slave owners and physicians forcing slaves in clinical testing. President Thomas Jefferson and Dr. J. Marion Sims were two prominent figures that used slaves in their research. Military experimentation conducted mustard gas experiments on African American, Hispanic, and Asian soldiers. Operation Big City piloted a program that spread different type of lung diseases in major cities. The Manhattan Project performed plutonium experiments on African Americans. Prison experimentation was influenced by Jim Crow medicine, which led to harmful tests in the Holmesburg Prison system.

Furthermore, black inmates endured marring experiments like the Sloan-Kettering Institute's cancer tests, the Kilby Draper and McAlester prisons' blood-plasma experiments, and Tulane University psycho-surgery experiments. Ironically, these experiments were conducted while international codes and ethical standards were implemented for clinical trials. By neglecting the process of informed consent, the experiments disregarded African Americans and other racial groups' autonomy, which violated the Nuremberg Code and the Declaration of Helsinki. In response to race-based experimentation, African Americans' developed an oral tradition of fear that resulted in black homeopathy. Black homeopathy became African Americans' medium of clinical justice to participate and be heard in the clinical process. Black homeopathy began the process of African Americans' reconciliation and contribution to medicine.

In Chapter 3, I examined American discourse of heart disease, the FDA's approval of BiDil, and biocapital, medicalization, biomedicalization and genetics' relation to race. The Framingham Heart Study set the precedence of pre-disposition illness testing of heart illness. The pathology of heart disease was understood by racial groups. White people were understood to have heart disease caused by neurasthenia. For most of the twentieth century, most of the cardiology community did not associate African Americans with having heart disease.

The Veterans Administration Cooperative Studies known as Vasodilator Heart Failure Trial (V-HeFT) I and II followed the Framingham Study. The elements of Hydralazine and Isosorbide dinitrate (H/I) were used in the V-HeFT I and II trials. The results of the trial concluded the H/I combination was efficacious in all groups, regardless of race. Cardiologist John Cohn seek to get the H/I combination approved by the FDA. Medco received patent rights to the H/I combination. The FDA denied approval due to unclear data. Cohn constructed the notion that H/I combination had a different effect on African Americans compared to other racial groups.

In Cohn's second attempt at approval, the FDA approved the H/I combination under findings of a race-based "distinction" in clinical trials. The findings were recorded in an article Cohn and Dr. Peter Carson wrote called "Racial Differences in Response to Therapy for Heart Failure: Analysis of the Vasodilator-Heart Failure Trials." The article promoted the African-American Heart Failure Trial (A-HeFT). The results of the trial were convincing enough for the FDA to approve the H/I combination to form the first race-based drug called BiDil.

Ultimately, the FDA had four justifications to approve BiDil. First, data from 3 clinical trials showed dramatic effectiveness of hydralazine hydrochloride and isosorbide dinitrate in black patients and supported a differential effect in black and white patients. Second, not understanding the reasons for the difference in treatment effect by race did not justify withholding the treatment from those who could benefit from it. Third, regulatory and other concerns associated with drug approval for narrow patient populations did not justify withholding BiDil from those who could benefit from it. Fourth, race and other demographic characteristics have long been important to consider in analysis of trials and as a matter of equity and justice.

The FDA's approval brought up many reservations because the data was misinterpreted and the H/I combination in African Americans produced ambiguous results. A huge reservation of BiDil's approval came from post hoc issues. Post hoc analyses of the two 1980s H/I trials were not exclusively from an African American population, but from the general population. The A-HeFT trial did not have another African American population as a control group. Lastly, the black–white ratio was omitted from NitroMed's study.

BiDil's approval raises many concerns because it suspiciously caused more questions than answers. The logic behind approving a drug that had an incomplete clinical process was for financial motives. The FDA approving a drug based on race created a lucrative drug market that targeted racial groups based on illness trends. As a result, race became a form of biocapital.

In relation to BiDil, NitroMed's role in biocapital constructed the notion of race to express an innovative technique for pharmacology and biotechnology. Like commercial capitalism, race is speculative in nature based on perception. For example, BiDil stock went up tremendously with its FDA approval, but when projections were bleak its stock fell. Financial motives influenced BiDil to have very poor funding and an impulsive clinical process. NitroMed tried to push BiDil into the black community through endorsements of prominent African American health groups like the Association of Black Cardiologists and the National Minority Health Month Foundation (NMHMF). Ultimately, BiDil was not successful because its price caused a financial disconnect for patient accessibility. BiDil cost more money than its competitors. Since there were alternatives that worked just as well or better than BiDil and cost substantially less, BiDil was not the prime choice for black patients. Most physicians did not prescribe BiDil because of it expensive cost and the racial claims it promotes.

From a legal perspective, the approval of BiDil was not compliant with the FFDC Act and the 1962 Amendments. The efficacy of BiDil for African Americans still was not clear. Also, the approval of BiDil influenced the medicalization & biomedicalization of race. Medicalization is the process when nonmedical issues become interpreted, defined, and treated as medical problems, usually labelled as a certain illness or disorder. In regard to heart illness and health inequity, medicalization is counterproductive because the problem is based on the individual and ignores social factors.

In BiDil's approval process, the chair of the FDA Advisory Committee Robert Nissen had poor examples of case studies that led to justifying BiDil's approval. Nissen's erroneous interpretation of case studies connected race with disease. His assertion reified race as a biological truth, which led to the FDA's justification that race was a proxy for disease. Nissen biomedicalized race by approving BiDil as a form of enhancing personalized medicine for the black community.

Biomedicalization used technoscience to produce identity through applying science and technology to our bodies which created identities and labels showed in BiDil. Racial notions imposed assumptions into one's sense of self and redefined new categories of health related identities. BiDil recreated the eugenic stratification of racial bodies as biologically different which draws inaccurate conclusions about disease pathology.

By the mid-twentieth century, UNESCO and other anthropological and sociological organizations confirmed race as 'myth.' Carl von Linnaeus and Johann Fredrich Blumenbach created the classification of skin color and racial categories which influenced the United States Office of Management and Budget and United States Patent and Trademark Office (PTO) incorporation of racial categories in American society. The racial categories were used as a means for biological research that supported the appropriation of race and biology in biomedicine. The OMB and PTO racial categories were used in international biobanks. Biobanks used classification which defined ethical choices that brought meaning and identification. The biobanks racial data was based out of the self-identification of individuals which was based on subjectivity. Self-identification does not have legitimate consensus among scientists and geneticists because it is not consistent with findings on the genetic level.

Genome-Wide Association Studies (GWAS) and EIGENSTRAT are technologies used in genetic variation and population. GWAS disease associations require methods for accounting for population differences. EIGENSTRAT is the type of technology that moves from genetic similarity, to genetic ancestry, to genome geography. Through GWAS and EIGENSTRAT, there was not genetic proof that African Americans are genetically different than other racial groups. Diseases like sickle cell anemia and cystic fibrosis have nothing to do with race, but a reality of geography, ancestry and recessive mutations in specific genes. Race-based medicine is not compatible with genetics and cause maleficence because one drug is not adequate to solve an entire racial groups' illness. Consequently, a race-based drug can cause Adverse Drug Reactions (ADRs) because the genetics of each individual can cause a different reaction to the drug.

Chapter 3 closes out with the examination of health inequity & discrimination acknowledging that race-based medicine cannot be an adequate solution to address these issues. I suggested solutions in the clinical setting by physicians perfecting their cultural competency, empathic communication, and awareness toward minority patients. Also, diet and nutrition is vital in improving health disparities in minority communities. When minority communities have equal access to healthy foods and nutrition education, the health inequity of minority communities can progressively decrease. Other health solutions in the black community are expressed through the black church's advocacy and its use of black theology.

Lastly, Chapter 4 discussed the black church's response to race-based medicine, allowing the voice of African Americans to be heard through health advocacy. Black theology was a tool to emphasize autonomy in minority communities by challenging concepts like polygenism that were attributed to scripture. Polygenism, coined by Paracelsus, was the belief humanity descended from two or more ancestral types. Polygenic claims were a result of misinterpretations of the book of Genesis.

By contrast, the Hebrew Scriptures and the New Testament had positive illustrations of black individuals. For example, Moses' Ethiopian wife and Simone of Cyrene were affirmative representations of blackness. Biblical narratives of the gospel of Mark were used as a tool to empower minority communities with their medical challenges. Finally, this chapter explored the past and present black church health advocacy movements and initiatives as substitutes to race-based medicine, and included a reflection on my personal efforts as a black clergyman.

Future Explorations

This book examined the history and relationship between race-based medicine and African Americans. Future research can examine the ways in which race-based medicine skews the perception about black bodies, and how such perceptions affect other social institutions, such as the criminal justice system and the beauty industry. Including other racial groups is significant; each racial group brings its unique experience to American medicine. More work is needed in discovering other racial groups' interaction with race-based medicine. On a global scale, future research can explore whether race-based medicine is relevant to homogenous countries. Lastly, in the wake of the Ebola and Zika virus outbreaks, analyzing race-based medicine could contribute to greater understanding about immigration debates and laws.

Bibliography

Agate, Lisa L., et al. "Churches United to Stop HIV (CUSH): A Faith-Based HIV Prevention Initiative." *Journal of the National Medical Association* 97, no. 7, Suppl. (2005), 60S.

Alexander, Denis, and Ronald L. Numbers. *Biology and Ideology from Descartes to Dawkins*. Chicago: University of Chicago Press, 2010.

Alter, Charlotte. "The HPV Vaccine and the Case for Race-Based Medicine." *Time Magazine*, November 11. Accessed on October 28, 2014. http://healthland.time.com/2013/11/01/the-hpv-vaccine-and-the-case-for-race-based-medicine/.

Aluoch, J. R. "Editorial: The Origin of the Sickle Cell Gene." *The East African Medical Journal: The Organ of the Medical Association of East Africa* 73, no. 9 (1996), 565.

Anderson, Warwick. "Teaching 'Race' at Medical School: Social Scientist on the Margin." *Social Studies of Science* 38, no. 5 (October 2008), 785–800. Sage.

Aronowitz, Robert A. *Making Sense of Illness: Science, Society, and Disease*. Cambridge, UK: Cambridge University Press, 1998.

Bader, Michael D. M., et al. "Disparities in Neighborhood Food Environments: Implications of Measurement Strategies." *Economic Geography* 86, no. 4 (October 2010).

© The Editor(s) (if applicable) and The Author(s) 2019
K. A. Johnson, *Medical Stigmata*,
https://doi.org/10.1007/978-981-13-2992-0

Bakalar, Nicholas. "Minorities Get Less Pain Treatment in E.R." *New York Times*, November 30, 2015. Accessed on December 2, 2015. http://well.blogs.nytimes.com/2015/11/30/minorities-get-less-pain-treatment-in-e-r/?ref=health&_r=0.

Balgir, R. S. "Indigenous and Independent Origin of the B*-Mutation in Ancient India: Is It a Myth Or Reality?" *Mankind Quarterly* 42, no. 2 (Winter 2001), 99–116.

Beauchamp, Tom, and James Childress. *Principles of Biomedical Ethics*, 6th ed. Oxford: Oxford University Press, 2008.

Bethencourt, Francisco. *Racisms: From the Crusades to the Twentieth Century*. Princeton: Princeton University Press, 2014.

Bell, Susan E., and Anne E. Figert. *Reimagining (Bio)Medicalization, Pharmaceuticals and Genetics: Old Critiques and New Engagements*. New York and Abingdon, Oxon: Routledge, 2015.

Birch, Kean, and David Tyfield. "Theorizing the Bioeconomy Biovalue, Biocapital, Bioeconomics or… What?" *Science, Technology & Human Values* 38, no. 3 (2013), 299–327.

Bliss, Catherine. *Race Decoded: The Genomic Fight for Social Justice*. Stanford, CA: Stanford University Press, 2012.

Booth, William. "Partnering with the Black Church: Recipe for Promoting Heart Health in the Stroke Belt." *ABNF Journal* 23, no. 2 (2012), 34–37.

Briggs, Charles L. "Communicability, Racial Discourse, and Disease." *Annual Review Anthropol* 34 (2005), 269–291.

Brodkin, Karen. *How Jews Became White Folks and What That Says About Race in America*. New Brunswick, NJ: Rutgers University Press, 1998.

Brody, Baruch A. *The Ethics of Biomedical Research: An International Perspective*. New York: Oxford University Press, 1998.

Brody, Howard, and Linda M. Hunt. "BiDil: Assessing a Race-Based Pharmaceutical." *Annals of Family Medicine* 4, no. 6 (November 1, 2006), 556–560.

Buckman, Robert, et al. "Empathic Responses in Clinical Practice: Intuition or Tuition?" *CMAJ: Canadian Medical Association Journal* 183, no. 5 (March 22, 2011).

Brown, Nancy. "Knowing Which Medical Products Are Best for Each Person—It Just Makes Sense." *The Huffington Post*, May 31. Accessed on May 31, 2014. http://www.huffingtonpost.com/nancy-brown/knowing-which-medical-pro_b_5044156.html.

Brown, Nancy. "CVGPS: Plotting the Best Route to Health for Each, Every Person." *The Huffington Post,* October 12. Accessed on October 28, 2014. http://www.huffingtonpost.com/nancy-brown/post_8211_b_5672360.html.

Cahill, Lisa Sowle. *Theological Bioethics.* Washington, DC: Georgetown University Press, 2005.

Campbell, Timothy, and Adam Sitze. *Biopolitics: A Reader.* Durham: Duke University Press, 2013.

Carey, Nessa. *The Epigenetics Revolution: How Modern Biology Is Rewriting Our Understanding of Genetics, Disease, and Inheritance.* New York: Columbia University Press, 2012.

CDC. "Statistical Policy Directive No. 15, Race and Ethnic Standards for Federal Statistics and Administrative Reporting." *CDC,* May 12, 1977. Accessed on August 20, 2015. http://wonder.cdc.gov/wonder/help/populations/bridged-race/directive15.html.

CDC. Community Health and Program Services (CHAPS): Health Disparities Among Racial/Ethnic Populations. Atlanta: US Department of Health and Human Services, 2008.

Chen, Xiang, and Xining Yang. "Does Food Environment Influence Food Choices? A Geographical Analysis Through 'Tweets'". *Applied Geography* 51 (2014), 82–89.

Clarke, Adele, et al. *Biomedicalization: Technoscience, Health, and Illness in the US.* Durham, NC: Duke University Press, 2010.

Cone, James. *A Black Theology of Liberation.* Philadelphia: Lippincott, 1970.

Conrad, Peter. *The Medicalization of Society: On the Transformation of Human Conditions into Treatable Disorders.* Baltimore: Johns Hopkins University Press, 2007.

Copher, Charles B., et al. *The Recovery of Black Presence: An Interdisciplinary Exploration: Essays in Honor of Dr. Charles B. Copher.* Nashville: Abingdon Press, 1995.

Cooper, Richard S., Jay S. Kaufman, and Ryk Ward. "Race and Genomics." *New England Journal of Medicine* 348, no. 12 (2003), 1166–1169.

Covey, Herbert C. *African American Slave Medicine: Herbal and Non-Herbal Treatments.* Lanham: Lexington Books, 2007.

Cox, John L. "Empathy, Identity and Engagement in Person-Centred Medicine: The Sociocultural Context." *Journal of Evaluation in Clinical Practice* 17, no. 2 (2011), 350–353.

Davis, Cynthia J. *Bodily and Narrative Forms: The Influence of Medicine on American Literature, 1845–1915.* Stanford, CA: Stanford University Press, 2000.

De La Torre, Miguel A. *Doing Christian Ethics from the Margins*. Maryknoll, NY: Orbis Books, 2004.

Dean, Wesley R., and Joseph R. Sharkey. "Rural and Urban Differences in the Associations Between Characteristics of the Community Food Environment and Fruit and Vegetable Intake." *Journal of Nutrition Education and Behavior* 43, no. 6 (2011), 426–433.

Downey, Laurence J. "BiDil: Alive and Kicking." *Lancet* 379, no. 9829 (May 19, 2012), 1876–1877.

Dressler, William W. "Health in the African American Community: Accounting for Health Inequalities." *Medical Anthropology Quarterly* 7, no. 4 (New Series). Racism, Gender, Class, and Health (December 1993), 325–345.

Dressler, William W., Kathryn S. Oths, and Clarence C. Gravlee. "Race and Ethnicity in Public Health Reasearch: Models to Explain Health Disparities." *Annual Review of Anthropology* 34 (October 2005), 231–252.

Duster, Troy. "Medicine, Culture, and Sickle Cell Disease." *The Hastings Center Report* 32, no. 4 (2002), 46–47.

Duster, Troy. *Backdoor to Eugenics*. New York: Routledge, 2003.

Duster, Troy. "Medicalisation of Race." *Lancet* 369, no. 9562 (February 24, 2007), 702–704.

Dych, William V. *Karl Rahner*. London: A&C Black, 2000.

El-Haj, Nadia Abu. "The Genetic Reinscription of Race." *Annual Review of Anthropology* 36 (2007), 283–300.

Epstein, Steven. "Bodily Differences and Collective Identities: The Politics of Gender and Race in Biomedical Research in the United States." *Body & Society* 10, no. 2/3 (June 2004), 183–203.

Epstein, Steven. *Inclusion: The Politics of Difference in Medical Research*. Chicago: University of Chicago Press, 2007.

FDA. "Understanding Investigational Drugs and Off Label Use of Approved Drugs." Last Modified June 24, 2015. http://www.fda.gov/ForPatients/Other/OffLabel/default.htm.

Felder, Cain Hope. *Stony the Road We Trod: African American Biblical Interpretation*. Minneapolis: Fortress Press, 1991.

Fett, Sharla M. *Working Cures: Healing, Health, and Power on Southern Slave Plantations*. Chapel Hill: University of North Carolina Press, 2002.

Foner, Nancy, and George M. Fredrickson. *Not Just Black and White: Historical and Contemporary Perspectives on Immigration, Race, and Ethnicity in the United States*. New York: Russell Sage Foundation, 2004.

Food & Drug Administration. "FDA Approves Treatment for Fat Below the Chin." *FDA*, April 29. Accessed on April 29, 2015. http://www.fda.gov/NewsEvents/Newsroom/PressAnnouncements/ucm444978.htm.

Foucault, Michel, and Michel Senellart. *The Birth of Biopolitics: Lectures at the Collège de France, 1978–1979*. Basingstoke, UK: Palgrave Macmillan, 2008.

Francis, Richard C. *Epigenetics: How Environment Shapes Our Genes*. New York: W. W. Norton, 2012.

Frank, Danielle, Thomas H. Gallagher, Sherrill L. Sellers, Lisa A. Cooper, Eboni G. Price, Adebola O. Odunlami, and Vence L. Bonham. "Primary Care Physicians Attitudes Regarding Race-Based Therapies." *JGIM: Journal of General Internal Medicine* 255, 384–389.

Franrenet, Sandra, et al. "Ethical Issues Related to Computerized Family Medical Histories in Sickle Cell Disease: Inforare." *Journal of Medical Ethics* 36, no. 10 (2010), 604.

Fujimura, Joan H., Troy Duster, Ramya Rajagopalan. "Introduction: Race, Genetics, and Disease: Questions of Evidence, Matters of Consequence." *Social Studies of Science* 38, no. 5 (October 2008), 643–656.

Fujimura, Joan H., and Ramya Rajagopalan. "Different Differences: The Use of 'Genetic Ancestry' Versus Race in Biomedical Human Genetic Research." *Social Studies of Science* 41, no. 1 (February 2011), 5–30.

Fullwiley, Duana. "The Biologistical Construction of Race: 'Admixture' Technology and the New Genetic Medicine." *Social Studies of Science* 38, no. 5 (October 2008), 695–735 (Sage Publications Ltd.).

Fuqua, Sonja R., et al. "Recruiting African-American Research Participation in the Jackson Heart Study: Methods, Response Rates, and Sample Description." *Ethn Dis* 15, no. 4 Suppl. 6 (2005), S6–18.

Gamble, Vanessa Northington. *Making a Place for Ourselves: The Black Hospital Movement, 1920–1945*. New York: Oxford University Press, 1995.

Gilman, Sander L. *Jewish Frontiers: Essays on Bodies, Histories, and Identities*. New York, NY: Palgrave Macmillan, 2003.

Goertzel, Ted George, and Ben Goertzel. *Linus Pauling: A Life in Science and Politics*. New York: Basic Books, 1995.

Goldschmidt, Debra. "FDA Approves New Cholesterol Lowering Drug." *CNN*, July 24. Accessed on July 24, 2015. http://www.cnn.com/2015/07/24/health/fda-cholesterol-drug-approved/index.html.

Grant, Jacquelyn. *White Women's Christ and Black Women's Jesus: Feminist Christology and Womanist Response*. Atlanta, GA: Scholars Press, 1989.

Graves, Joseph L. *The Emperor's New Clothes: Biological Theories of Race at the Millennium*. New Brunswick, NJ: Rutgers University Press, 2001.

Gravlee, Clarence C. "How Race Becomes Biology: Embodiment of Social Inequality." *American Journal of Physical Anthropology* 139, no. 1 (May 2009), 47–57.

Gunderson, Gary, and James R. Cochrane. *Religion and the Health of the Public: Shifting the Paradigm*. New York: Palgrave Macmillan, 2012.

Gunn, D. M., and Danna Nolan Fewell. *Narrative in the Hebrew Bible*. New York: Oxford University Press, 1993.

Hager, Thomas. *Force of Nature: The Life of Linus Pauling*. New York: Simon & Schuster, 1995.

Hansen, Randall, and Desmond S. King. *Sterilized by the State: Eugenics, Race, and the Population Scare in Twentieth-Century North America*. New York: Cambridge University Press, 2013.

Hart, Mitchell B. "Racial Science, Social Science, and the Politics of Jewish Assimilation." *Isis* (1999), 268–297.

Hawkins-Taylor, Chamika, and Angeline M. Carlson. "Communication Strategies Must Be Tailored to a Medication's Targeted Population: Lessons from the Case of BiDil." *American Health & Drug Benefits* 6, no. 7 (2013), 401.

Henderson, Carol E. *Imagining the Black Female Body: Reconciling Image in Print and Visual Culture*. New York: Palgrave Macmillan, 2010.

Hoberman, John M. *Darwin's Athletes: How Sport Has Damaged Black America and Preserved the Myth of Race*. Boston: Houghton Mifflin, 1997.

Holliday, R. *Epigenetics: A Historical Overview*. London: Henry Stewart Talks, 2007.

Holloway, Karla F. C. *Private Bodies, Public Texts: Race, Gender, and a Cultural Bioethics*. Durham, NC: Duke University Press, 2011.

Hopkins, Dwight N. *Down, Up, and Over: Slave Religion and Black Theology*. Minneapolis, MN: Fortress Press, 2000.

Hornblum, Allen M. *Acres of Skin: Human Experiments at Holmesburg Prison : A Story of Abuse and Exploitation in the Name of Medical Science*. New York: Routledge, 1998.

Houser, Heather. *Ecosickness in Contemporary US Fiction: Environment and Affect*, 2014.

Inda, Jonathan Xavier. "For Blacks Only: Pharmaceuticals, Genetics, and the Racial Politics of Life." *Materiali Foucaultiani* 1, no. 2 (2012), 107–135.

"Illuminating BiDil." *Nature Biotechnology* 23, no. 8 (August 2005), 903.

Jackson, Ronald L. *Scripting the Black Masculine Body Identity, Discourse, and Racial Politics in Popular Media.* Albany: State University of New York Press, 2006.

Johnson, Sylvester A. *The Myth of Ham in Nineteenth-Century American Christianity: Race, Heathens, and the People of God.* New York: Palgrave Macmillan, 2004.

Johnson, Kirk, et. al. "Rachel Dolezal, in Center of Storm, Is Defiant: 'I Identify as Black.'" *New York Times,* June 16, 2015. Accessed on July 7, 2015. http://www.nytimes.com/2015/06/17/us/rachel-dolezal-nbc-today-show.html.

Kahn, Jonathan. "Exploiting Race in Drug Development: BiDil's Interim Model of Pharmacogenomics." *Social Studies of Science* 38, no. 5 (October 2008), 737–758 (Sage Publications Ltd.).

Kahn, Jonathan D., et al. "Flaws in the US Food and Drug Administration's Rationale for Supporting the Development and Approval of BiDil as a Treatment for Heart Failure Only in Black Patients." *Journal of Law, Medicine & Ethics* 36, no. 3 (Fall 2008), 449–457.

Kahn, Jonathan. *Race in a Bottle: The Story of BiDil and Racialized Medicine in a Post-Genomic Age.* New York: Columbia University Press, 2013.

Kirsh, Nurit. "Population Genetics in Israel in the 1950s: The Unconscious Internalization of Ideology." *Isis* 94, no. 4 (2003), 631–655.

Krimsky, Sheldon. "The Art of Medicine: The Short Life of a Race Drug." *Lancet* 379, no. 9811 (January 14, 2012), 114–115.

LaMotte, Sandee. "Health Effects of Coffee: Where Do We Stand?" *CNN,* August 14, 2015. Accessed on August 16, 2015. http://www.cnn.com/2015/08/14/health/coffee-health/index.html.

Largent, Mark A. *Breeding Contempt: The History of Coerced Sterilization in the United States.* New Brunswick, NJ: Rutgers University Press, 2008.

Lee, Sandra Soo-Jin. "Health Policy and Ethics. Racializing Drug Design: Implications of Pharmacogenomics for Health Disparities." *American Journal of Public Health* 95, no. 12 (December 2005), 2133–2138.

Lee, Sandra Soo-Jin, and Ashwin Mudaliar. "Racing Forward: The Genomics and Personalized Medicine Act." *Science* 323, no. 5912 (January 16, 2009), 342.

Lemke, Thomas. *Biopolitics: An Advanced Introduction.* New York: New York University Press, 2011.

Livingstone, David N. *Adam's Ancestors: Race, Religion, and the Politics of Human Origins.* Baltimore: Johns Hopkins University Press, 2008.

Luhby, Tami. "5 Disturbing Stats on Black-White Inequality." *CNN,* August 21, 2014. Accessed on July 18, 2015. http://money.cnn.com/2014/08/21/news/economy/black-white-inequality/.

Lysaught, M. Therese. *On Moral Medicine: Theological Perspectives in Medical Ethics*. Grand Rapids, Mich: W. B. Eerdmans, 2012.

"Malpractice." *Encyclopedia Britannica Inc.* Web, November 10, 2014. http://www.britannica.com.ezproxy.drew.edu/EBchecked/topic/360514/malpractice.

Markel, Howard. *Quarantine! East European Jewish Immigrants and the New York City Epidemics of 1892*. Baltimore, MD: Johns Hopkins University Press, 1997.

Markel, Howard. *When Germs Travel: Six Major Epidemics That Have Invaded America Since 1900 and the Fears They Have Unleashed*. New York: Pantheon Books, 2004.

Mays, Vickie M., Susan D. Cochran, and W. Barne, Namdi. "Race, Race-Based Discrimination, and Health Outcomes Among African Americans." *Annual Review of Psychology* 58 (January 2007), 201–225.

McBride, David. *From TB to AIDS: Epidemics Among Urban Blacks Since 1900*. Albany: State University of New York Press, 1991.

McKnight, Whitney. *Infectious Disease News* 24, no. 6 (June 2011).

Meier, Robert J. "A Critique of Race-Based and Genomic Medicine." *Collegium Antropologicum* 36, no. 1 (March 2012), 5–10.

Moreno, Jonathan D. *Undue Risk: Secret State Experiments on Humans*. New York: W. H. Freeman, 2000.

Mugalu, Joachim. *Philosophy, Oral Tradition and Africanistics: A Survey of the Aesthetic and Cultural Aspects of Myth, with a Case-Study of the "Story of Kintu" from Buganda (Uganda), as a Contribution to the Philosophical Investigations in Oral Traditions*. Frankfurt am Main: Peter Lang, 1995.

Nelson, Alondra. *Body and Soul: The Black Panther Party and the Fight Against Medical Discrimination*. Minneapolis: University of Minnesota Press, 2011.

Neuwirth, Zeev E. "Physician Empathy—Should We Care?" *The Lancet* 350, no. 9078 (August 30, 1997).

Nolen, Claude H. *The Negro's Image in the South: The Anatomy of White Supremacy*. Lexington: University of Kentucky Press, 1967.

Oikkonen, Venla. "Mitochondrial Eve and the Affective Politics of Human Ancestry." *Signs* 40, no. 3 (2015), 747–772.

Parrington, John. *The Deeper Genome: Why There Is More to the Human Genome Than Meets the Eye*, 2015.

Pauling, Linus, Clifford Mead, and Thomas Hager. *Linus Pauling: Scientist and Peacemaker*. Corvallis: Oregon State University Press, 2001.

Payne, Thomas J., et al. "Sociocultural Methods in the Jackson Heart Study: Conceptual and Descriptive Overview." *Ethn Dis* 15, no. Suppl. 6 (2005), S6-38.

Peterson, Eric, and Clyde W. Yancy. "Eliminating Racial and Ethnic Disparities in Cardiac Care." *New England Journal of Medicine* 360, no. 12 (2009), 1172–1174.

Pinn, Anthony B. *The Black Church in the Post-Civil Rights Era*. Maryknoll, NY: Orbis Books, 2002.

Pollock, Anne. *Medicating Race: Heart Disease and Durable Preoccupations with Difference*. Durham: Duke University Press, 2012.

Prograis, Lawrence, and Edmund D. Pellegrino. *African American Bioethics: Culture, Race, and Identity*. Washington, DC: Georgetown University Press, 2007.

Quinn, Sandra Crouse, and Stephen B. Thomas. "The National Negro Health Week, 1915 to 1951: A Descriptive Account." *Minority Health Today* 2, no. 3 (2001), 44–49.

Reuter, Shelley Z. "The Genuine Jewish Type: Racial Ideology and Anti-Immigrationism in Early Medical Writing About Tay-Sachs Disease." *Canadian Journal of Sociology* 31, no. 3 (Summer 2006), 291–323.

Roberts, Dorothy E. *Fatal Invention: How Science, Politics, and Big Business Re-Create Race in the Twenty-First Century*. New York: New Press, 2011.

Rose, Nikolas S. *Politics of Life Itself: Biomedicine, Power, and Subjectivity in the Twenty-First Century*. Princeton: Princeton University Press, 2007.

Rodriguez, Judith C. "Serving the Public: Health Literacy and Food Deserts." *Journal of the American Dietetic Association* 111, no. 1 (2011), 14.

Rund, D., et al. "The Origin of Sickle Cell Alleles in Israel." *Human Genetics* 85, no. 5 (1990), 521–524.

Sadler, Rodney S. "Can A Cushite Change His Skin? Cushites, 'Racial Othering' and the Hebrew Bible." *Interpretation* 60, no. 4 (2006), 386–403.

Santoro, Michael A., and Thomas M. Gorrie. *Ethics and the Pharmaceutical Industry*. Cambridge: Cambridge University Press, 2005.

Savitt, Todd Lee. *Race and Medicine in Nineteenth- and Early-Twentieth-Century America*. Kent, OH: Kent State University Press, 2007.

Schrag, Peter. *Not Fit for Our Society: Nativism and Immigration*. Berkeley: University of California Press, 2010.

Schwartz, Robert S. "Racial Profiling in Medical Research." *The New England Journal of Medicine* 344, no. 18 (May 3, 2001), 1392–1393.

Schwartz, Pamela Yew. "Why Is Neurasthenia Important in Asian Cultures?" *Western Journal of Medicine* 176, no. 4 (2002), 257–258.

Shim, Janet K. "Constructing 'Race' Across the Science-Lay Divide: Racial Formation in the Epidemiology and Experience of Cardiovascular Disease." *Social Studies of Science* 35, no. 3 (June 2005), 405–436.

Shim, Janet K. *Heart-Sick: The Politics of Risk, Inequality, and Heart Disease.* New York and London: New York University Press, 2014.

Shin, Laura. "The Racial Wealth Gap: Why a Typical White Household Has 16 Times the Wealth of a Black One." *Forbes*, March 26, 2015. Accessed on July 18, 2015. http://www.forbes.com/sites/laurashin/2015/03/26/the-racial-wealth-gap-why-a-typical-white-household-has-16-times-the-wealth-of-a-black-one/.

Smedley, Brian D., Adrienne Y. Stith, and Alan R. Nelson. *Unequal Treatment: Confronting Racial and Ethnic Disparities in Health Care.* Washington, DC: National Academy Press, 2003.

Smith, Susan L. *Sick and Tired of Being Sick and Tired: Black Women's Health Activism in America, 1890–1950.* Philadelphia: University of Pennsylvania Press, 1995.

Smith, Susan L. "Mustard Gas and American Race-Based Human Experimentation in World War II." *The Journal of Law, Medicine & Ethics* 36, no. 3 (2008), 517–521.

Sohi, Inderbir, et al. "Differences in Food Environment Perceptions and Spatial Attributes of Food Shopping Between Residents of Low and High Food Access Areas." *Journal of Nutrition Education and Behavior* 46, no. 4 (2014), 241–249.

Steinbock, Bonnie. *The Oxford Handbook of Bioethics.* Oxford: Oxford University Press, 2007.

Stern, Alexandra. *Eugenic Nation: Faults and Frontiers of Better Breeding in Modern America.* Berkeley: University of California Press, 2005.

Stith, Richard. "Toward Freedom from Value." *The Jurist* 38 (1978).

Stoneking, Mark, Rebecca L. Cann, and Allan C. Wilson. "Mitochondrial DNA and Human Evolution." *Nature* 325 (6099) (1987), 31–36.

Sunder Rajan, Kaushik. *Biocapital: The Constitution of Postgenomic Life.* Durham: Duke University Press, 2006.

Sussman, Robert W. *The Myth of Race: The Troubling Persistence of an Unscientific Idea.* Cambridge: Harvard University Press, 2014.

Taylor, Ann L., et. al. "The African-American Heart Failure Trial: Background, Rationale and Significance." *Journal of the National Medical Association* 94, no. 9 (September 2002), 762–769.

Taylor, Henry A., Jr. "The Jackson Heart Study: An Overview." *Ethn Dis* 15 (Autumn 2005) (4 Suppl. 6), S6-1-3.

Tapper, Melbourne. *In the Blood: Sickle Cell Anemia and the Politics of Race.* Philadelphia: University of Pennsylvania Press, 1999.

Tapper, Melbourne. "Interrogating Bodies: Medico-Racial Knowledge, Politics, and the Study of a Disease." *Comparative Studies in Society & History* 37, no. 1 (January 1995), 76–93.

Tattersall, Ian, and Rob DeSalle. *Race? Debunking a Scientific Myth.* College Station: Texas A&M University Press, 2011.

Temple, Robert, and Norman L. Stockbridge. "BiDil for Heart Failure in Black Patients: The US Food and Drug Administration Perspective." *Annals of Internal Medicine* 146, no. 1 (January 2, 2007), 57-W9.

Townes, Emilie Maureen. *Breaking the Fine Rain of Death: African American Health Issues and a Womanist Ethic of Care.* New York: Continuum, 1998.

Vatter, Miguel. *The Republic of the Living: Biopolitics and the Critique of Civil Society.* Fordham University Press, 2014.

Verhey, Allen. *Reading the Bible in the Strange World of Medicine.* Grand Rapids, Mich: W. B. Eerdmans, 2003.

Vigen, Aana Marie. *Women, Ethics, and Inequality in US Healthcare: "To Count Among the Living."* New York: Palgrave Macmillan, 2006.

Wailoo, Keith. *Drawing Blood: Technology and Disease Identity in Twentieth-Century America.* Baltimore: Johns Hopkins University Press, 1997.

Wailoo, Keith. *Dying in the City of the Blues: Sickle Cell Anemia and the Politics of Race and Health.* Chapel Hill: University of North Carolina Press, 2001.

Wailoo, Keith, Alondra Nelson, and Catherine Lee. *Genetics and the Unsettled Past: The Collision of DNA, Race, and History.* New Brunswick, NJ: Rutgers University Press, 2012.

Wailoo, Keith, and Stephen Gregory Pemberton. *The Troubled Dream of Genetic Medicine: Ethnicity and Innovation in Tay-Sachs, Cystic Fibrosis, and Sickle Cell Disease.* Baltimore: Johns Hopkins University Press, 2006.

Wald, Priscilla. *Contagious: Cultures, Carriers, and the Outbreak Narrative.* Durham: Duke University Press, 2008.

Walker, Renee E., et al. "Disparities and Access to Healthy Food in the United States: A Review of Food Deserts Literature." *Health & Place* 16, no. 5 (September 2010), 876–884.

Washington, Harriet A. *Medical Apartheid: The Dark History of Medical Experimentation on Black Americans from Colonial Times to the Present.* New York: Doubleday, 2006.

Weems, Renita J. *Just a Sister Away: A Womanist Vision of Women's Relationships in the Bible*. San Diego, CA: LuraMedia, 1988.

Welsome, Eileen. *The Plutonium Files: America's Secret Medical Experiments in the Cold War*. New York, NY: Dial Press, 1999.

West, Cornel. *Race Matters*. New York: Vintage Books, 1994.

White, Augustus A., and David Chanoff. *Seeing Patients: Unconscious Bias in Health Care*. Cambridge, MA: Harvard University Press, 2011.

Whitmarsh, Ian, and David S. Jones. *What's the Use of Race? Modern Governance and the Biology of Difference*. Cambridge, MA: MIT Press, 2010.

Widener, Michael J., et al. "Dynamic Urban Food Environments: A Temporal Analysis of Access to Healthy Foods." *American Journal of Preventive Medicine* 41, no. 4 (October 2011), 439–441.

Williams, Delores S. *Sisters in the Wilderness: The Challenge of Womanist God-Talk*. Maryknoll, NY: Orbis Books, 1993.

Wogaman, J. Philip, Douglas M. Strong, and J. Philip Wogaman. *Readings in Christian Ethics: A Historical Sourcebook*. Louisville, KY: Westminster John Knox Press, 1996.

Yudell, Michael. *Race Unmasked: Biology and Race in the Twentieth Century*. New York: Columbia University Press, 2014.

Zack, Naomi. *Philosophy of Science and Race*. New York: Routledge, 2002.

Zarcadoolas, Christina, Andrew F. Pleasant, and David S. Greer. *Advancing Health Literacy: A Framework for Understanding and Action*. San Francisco, CA: Jossey-Bass, 2006.

Printed in the USA
CPSIA information can be obtained
at www.ICGtesting.com
LVHW020627271123
764912LV00004B/161